Chiari Malformat Treatments

By John Hewitt, M.A,

Edited by Michelle Gabata, M.D.

CUTCHOGUE - NEW SUFFOLK
FREE LIBRARY

Editor in Chief: Michelle Gabata, M.D.

© 2011 John Hewitt, MA, Michelle Gabata MD

All Rights Reserved worldwide under the Berne Convention. May not be copied or distributed without prior written permission by the publisher. If you have this book or an electronic document and didn't pay for it, then the author didn't get a fair share. Please consider paying for your copy by purchasing it at any bookstore. Thank you!

Printed in the United States of America

ISBN: 1453895442

Contents

One: What is Chiari Malformation? 4

Two: Classification 8

Three: Causes 12

Four: Symptoms 14

Five: Diagnosis 20

Six: Treatment 22

Seven: Research & Studies 29

Eight: Brain Structure 36

Nine: Tests 43

Ten: What to Expect from Brain Surgery 53

Eleven: A Genetics Primer 60

Glossary of Medical Terms 106

Appendix A: Internet Resources / Further Reading 126

One: What is Chiari Malformation?

Chiari Malformation is a rare condition that was first described in 1891 by Hans von Chiari, a pathologist ; it is characterized by structural defects in the cerebellum, the bottom region of the brain that's in charge of controlling your body's balance and coordination. This rather complex condition occurs when your cerebellum and your brain stem (the back-end region of your brain), are pushed downwards through the foramen magnum, an opening located at the lower back end of the skull.

To better understand Chiari Malformation, it's necessary to explain some details of your body's anatomy. Your cerebellum controls your body's balance and coordination of motion; it is located at the base of your skull, also referred to as the posterior fossa. The cerebellum is made up of two lateral halves, or hemispheres. Underneath these hemispheres, there are two small protrusions called cerebellar tonsils. Normally, all of these sit on top of the foramen magnum, the opening located at the base of the skull through which the brain stem comes out and connects to the spinal cord. Your brain stem is involved in functions like respiratory control, pain sensitivity control, sleep cycle, and consciousness.

If your skull happens to be abnormally small or misshapen, it can press on your brain and force it downwards leading to the displacement of your cerebellum and your brain stem towards the foramen magnum and into the upper spinal canal. This is also referred to as cerebellar herniation. When this happens, your cerebellum and your spinal cord are placed under great pressure, and the flow of the cerebrospinal fluid (a clear liquid that covers and cushions your brain and your spinal cord) gets obstructed. This, in turn, will eventually result in the blockage of the signals that are transmitted by your brain to your body as well as the buildup of spinal fluid in the spinal cord. As a result, certain body functions will be affected. In addition, the pressure exerted on your spinal cord may lead to the development of neurological signs or symptoms.

Depending on the severity of the condition, you may not experience any symptoms at all, or you may experience a wide range of symptoms including dizziness, muscle weakness, numbness, chronic fatigue, vision problems, headaches, and balance and coordination problems. In the most severe cases, complete or partial paralysis of the body may occur as a result of the pressure built up on the spinal cord. Paralysis is usually permanent and can't be treated with surgery.

In most cases, Chiari Malformation has been identified to be congenital, meaning that it is present at birth. However, acquired cases of this disease have also been observed as a result of inherited disorders such as excessive joint mobility (in the case of of Ehlers-Danlos syndrome) and connective tissue weakness (Marfan Syndrome).

Due to the fact that a genetic prevalence was identified in some families, researchers continue to investigate the genetic implications of this condition and continue to search for the gene that may be responsible for causing it. In the past, Chiari Malformation was estimated to occur in about one in every 1,000 births. However, more recently it's been shown that this condition may actually be much more common. It's also been observed that Chiari Malformation occurs more often in women than in men. Getting an accurate estimate of the prevalence of this condition is complicated since some children that are born with it may not show any symptoms until adolescence or adulthood, if at all. In addition, because symptoms can often resemble those of other conditions, the malformation is frequently misdiagnosed.

Two: Classification

Chiari Malformations have been classified into four main types according to the severity of the disorder and the parts of the brain that protrude into the spinal canal.

Type I: This is the most common type of Chiari Malformation, and it's the only type that can also be acquired. It occurs when the lower part of your cerebellum is pushed into the foramen magnum without involving the brain stem. Many patients with Type I Chiari don't present any symptoms; when symptoms are present, usually headaches, they don't appear until adolescence or early adulthood. Symptoms very rarely present in young children. It's for these reasons that Type I Chiari Malformation often goes unnoticed and tends to be diagnosed by accident during the examination for another condition. Type I Chiari Malformation is often associated with anomalies in the base of the skull and the spine including curvatures of the spine, union of the first level of the spine to the base of the skull, and Klippel-Feil deformity, which is the fusion of levels of the spine within the neck.

Type II: This type, also known as Classic Chiari Malformation or Arnold-Chiari Malformation, occurs when both the cerebellum and the brain stem are pushed through the opening of the foramen magnum. In some cases, the cerebellar vermis, the nerve tissue that links the two halves of the cerebellum, may be only partially present or may even be absent. Type II patients often present meningomyelocoele, a birth defect that occurs when the spinal canal and the backbone don't close before birth. Normally, the two sides of the spine, or the backbone, join together and close, covering the spinal cord and its nerves. Meningomyelocoele causes the spinal cord and its protective membrane to stick out of the back. As a result, it can cause partial or complete paralysis in the legs and sometimes in the arms. It's been observed that about a third of the patients that present meningomyelocoele develop brain stem dysfunctions by the age of five, and a third of them die in infancy. Cranial nerve and brain stem dysfunctions are the most serious features of Type II Chiari Malformation.

Type III: Although very uncommon, this is the most serious type as it can cause severe neurological defects. It occurs when the cerebellum and the brain stem protrude through the foramen magnum opening into the spinal cord. In addition, in this type of Chiari Malformation, some parts of the brain's fourth ventricle (a cavity filled with cerebrospinal fluid that links the upper parts of the brain) can also stick out through the foramen magnum opening into the spinal cord. In some rare cases, it can lead to an occipital encephalocele, which is a sac-shaped structure containing brain matter that sticks out from the back of the head or the neck. Infants with type III Chiari malformation may suffer life threatening complications.

Type IV: This is a rather rare type of Chiari Malformation that involves cerebellar hypoplasia, an incomplete or underdeveloped cerebellum. As a matter of fact, in this type of malformation, parts of the cerebellum are often missing.

An additional type of Chiari Malformation has been suggested, which is type 0. In this type, some scientists are still contesting, there's no displacement of the cerebellum below the foramen magnum opening, but the patients present signs of Chiari Malformation including frequent headaches and the formation of a syrinx—a fluid cavity in the spinal cord.

Three: Causes

In most cases, Chiari Malformation has been identified to be present at birth. The exact mechanism that leads to this disorder hasn't been determined yet, but it has been observed that this disorder can result from several different causes. First, it's hypothesized that problems during the development of the fetus can lead to the abnormal formation of the brain. Factors such as the exposure to harmful substances or chemicals, drug and alcohol consumption, the lack of proper vitamins and nutrients in the diet, and other infections during pregnancy can predispose the fetus to problems that hinder the normal development of its head. As a result, the baby may develop structural defects in the cerebellum, the spinal cord, and the brain stem. Genetic mutations during fetal development can also lead to the Chiari Malformation. The cause for such genetic mutations still remains a mystery.

In some cases, a genetic prevalence of the condition has been observed. Therefore, studies are continuously carried out to find more about the genetic implications of this condition and to search for the gene that may be responsible for its development. Additionally, this condition can be acquired, meaning that it can be caused later in life by external factors. This is termed as Secondary Chiari Malformation and happens if spinal fluid is drained excessively from the spine as a result of injury, exposure to harmful or toxic substances, or infections. In some rare cases, high pressure in the brain compartment can exert downwards pressure on the cerebellum. Primary Chiary malformation is more common than the secondary type.

Four: Symptoms

The symptoms presented by the patients will vary depending on the type of Chiari Malformation that they suffer and the extent of the condition.

In the case of type I Chiari Malformation, a lot of patients don't have any symptoms. As a matter of fact, you may not even know that you have this type of condition. It is for this reason that type I is often diagnosed by accident while treating for other conditions. Even though a large number of type I patients usually don't present any symptoms, there are also patients that show symptoms like neck pains, overall weakness, poor hand coordination, balance or coordination problems, and headaches in the back of the head that worsen when coughing, running laughing or straining. Additional symptoms like vision problems, ringing in the ears, and vomiting have also been observed in type I patients. When these symptoms are present, they are often vague or nonspecific leading to misdiagnosis.

The symptoms of the other types of Chiari Malformation are more visible than those of Type I, and they tend to develop earlier. In the case of babies, some of the symptoms that have been observed include difficulty in swallowing, irritability when being fed, excessive drooling, vomiting, neck stiffness, breathing problems, arm weakness, and other developmental delays. In adults, the symptoms that you may present include headaches, numbness or weakness in the arms and legs, dizziness, and ear buzzing. You may also notice vision problems such as involuntary eye movements or double or blurred vision. In addition, balance and coordination problems are common resulting to occasions of vertigo or dizziness. You may experience difficulties while bending over, lifting heavy objects, standing or sitting for a long period of time, and engaging in strenuous activities like sports. In severe cases, Chiari Malformation can lead to the compression of the cranial nerve, which in turn can cause the cessation of breathing.

Besides the above listed symptoms, it's been observed that patients who suffer from Chiari Malformation often present the following related conditions:

Spinal curvature: This condition can be observed in patients with Type I Chiari Malformation. There are two types of spinal curvature: scoliosis and kyphosis. Scoliosis is produced when the spine is bent sideways, either to the left or to the right. Kyphosis, on the other hand, results when the spine is bent forwards. Spinal curvature is more common in children with Chiari Malformation than in adults because their bones have not been fully formed yet.

Hydrocephalus: In many cases, Chiari Malformation blocks the regular flow of the cerebrospinal fluid to the brain, causing excessive buildup of the fluid. This condition is known as hydrocephalus, and it causes pressure within the head that can lead to mental deficiencies and/or an enlarged skull. Severe hydrocephalus can be fatal if it's not properly treated. Although this condition can occur in any type of Chiari Malformation, it's more often observed in type II patients.

Spina bifida: This condition refers to the incomplete development of the spinal cord or its protective covering. Due to the fact that the bones around the spinal cord don't form and close properly before birth, part of the cord is left exposed. As a result, partial or complete paralysis can occur below the spinal defect. Individuals with Type II Chiari Malformation usually have myelomeningocele, which is a type of spina bifida in which the bones of the back and the lower spine don't form properly and extend out of the back in an opening that resembles a sac.

Syringomyelia: Also known as hydromyelia, this is a condition in which a syrinx (a sort of cyst that's filled with cerebrospinal fluid) forms in the central canal of the spinal cord. As the syrinx grows larger, it destroys the center of the spinal cord, causing pain, weakness, and rigidity in the back, neck, shoulders, arms, or legs. Additional symptoms that can be observed with syringomyelia include headaches and the loss of feeling of extreme temperatures, whether hot or cold, particularly in the hands. Syringomyelia can arise as a complication of other conditions such as trauma, meningitis, or tumors. There have also been cases in which this condition was present at birth. It's been shown that Chiari Malformation is its leading cause although the direct link is still not fully understood. It's hypothesized that it's related to the interference of the normal cerebrospinal flow caused by the obstruction of a part of the cerebellum at the foramen magnum.

Tethered cord syndrome: This is a progressive disorder that occurs when the spinal cord attaches itself to the spine bone, causing the spinal cord to stretch. This, in turn, can lead to permanent damage to the muscles and nerves in the lower body. It's been observed that children who have myelomeningocele, a birth defect that occurs when the spinal canal and the backbone don't close before birth, have a higher risk of developing a tethered cord syndrome later in life.

If you have any family history of Chiari Malformation or if you present any of the symptoms that are listed above, it's very important for you to talk to your doctor as soon as possible to carry out the proper tests. Early diagnosis is essential for the adequate treatment of the symptoms and prevention of other complications.

Five: Diagnosis

A lot of people with Chiari Malformation are asymptomatic, meaning they don't have any symptoms, and their condition is found out during the diagnosis or treatment for another disorder. However, if this condition occurs simultaneously with other defects that are present at birth, the diagnosis may be made right away at birth. Prenatal screenings with ultrasounds can also be used to diagnose the disease even before the birth of the baby.

In most cases, your doctor will carry out some tests after the onset of specific signs and symptoms to make a diagnosis. During the process of diagnosis, the doctor will most likely begin by evaluating your previous medical records and asking about your family's medical history. Your doctor will then proceed with a physical exam. He or she may also check some of the skills and functions that are related to your cerebellum like your memory, touch, reflexes, balance and coordination and other motor skills.

In addition, your doctor may also order one or several of the following tests to confirm the diagnosis of Chiari Malformations:

Magnetic resonance imaging (MRI)

X-rays

3D Computed tomography (CT scan) and Cine Imaging (Movie of the brain)

Brain stem auditory evoked potential (BAER)

Myleogram

Somatosensory Evoked Potentials (SSEP)

In some cases, the diagnosis of Chiari Malformation may be delayed or missed because some patients don't show any symptoms and also because the symptoms of this condition can mimic those of other more common disorders like migraine headaches, multiple sclerosis, and brain tumors.

Six: Treatment

The treatment depends on a case by case basis. Your doctor will make the appropriate recommendations after having evaluated the type of Chiari Malformation that you have, its progression as well as the symptoms that you present.

In some cases, particularly in many patients with type I Chiari Malformation, the symptoms may be mild and may not be progressive. It could even be the case that you're completely asymptotic, meaning that you don't have any symptoms. In such cases, your doctor may recommend you to follow a conservative management treatment process. As part of this process, your doctor may prescribe you some medications to help you manage and ease symptoms such as headache and pains. He or she may also suggest some physical therapy to help with the treatment. It has been reported that some patients have opted to explore non-traditional options like herbal therapy and acupuncture to treat this condition. Before deciding to follow any of these types of options, you should make sure to consult with your doctor. It's important that you take measures to minimize neck strain during the day and even when you sleep. In addition, it's recommended that you avoid chiropractic manipulations since you'll run the risk of aggravating your condition.

In more severe cases, your doctor may recommend a surgical operation. Surgery, in fact, is the only treatment available to some extent correct the functional injuries and to stop the progression of damage to the central nervous system. There are a number of different surgical procedures available to treat Chiari Malformation and any of the other conditions that may arise as a result of this disorder.

The most commonly used procedure is called decompression of the posterior fossa, which is the back of your skull. On the day of the surgery, you'll be administered with general anesthesia to put you asleep, and you'll be placed lying face down on the operating table. Then, an antiseptic will be applied in the surgical area, and the surgeon will make a small incision through your neck muscles to take a look at your skull and the top of your spine. Afterwards, the surgeon will perform a craniectomy, which consists of removing a small section of your skull bones (In other cases, removal of a part of the spinal column is necessary) . By doing so, he or she will be able to create more space in the back of your head, and the pressure on your cerebellum and brain stem will be reduced. That way, these two regions of the brain will be able to go back to their normal anatomical positions, the pressure on the spinal cord will be relieved, and the normal flow of the cerebrospinal fluid will be restored. After the surgery, you'll need a recovery period. Some of the typical post-surgery symptoms include headaches and neck pain that can last for several days.

In some cases, your surgeon may decide to take an additional step to make an incision in the dura, the covering part of the brain, to have a better view of your brain and your spinal cord. Then, the surgeon may add extra tissue to the dura to create more space to allow for the proper flow of cerebrospinal fluid.

Another procedure called spinal laminectomy may be performed. This procedure involves the surgical removal of part of your lamina (the arched roof of the spinal canal) to increase the size of the spinal canal, relieving pressure on the spinal cord and the nerve roots. Electrocautery is used sometimes by surgeons to decrease the size of your cerebellar tonsils, two small protrusions located on the bottom region of your cerebellum. In this procedure, tissues are eliminated using high-frequency electrical currents.

If you have hydrocephalus, or excessive buildup of cerebrospinal fluid, your surgeon may decide to treat this with a shunt system, a method by which a tube is inserted in your brain to drain the fluids into the abdominal cavity or chest wall. Another alternative surgical procedure is third ventriculostomy, a surgical operation that improves CSF flow by creating a small perforation in the floor of the third ventricle to divert CSF into the subarachnoid space thus relieving pressure.

Syringomyelia, a sort of cyst that's filled with cerebrospinal fluid and that forms in the central canal of the spinal cord, can be treated by inserting a small tube in the spinal cord for drainage.

Many Chiari Malformation patients who received surgery saw a reduction in their signs and symptoms, especially in the case of infant patients. While precise data is not available, it's estimated that about 50% of patients became symptom free after surgery, another 20%-30% improved significantly, and about 20% experienced no relief or got worse.

During the first 24 hours after surgery, you'll be under observation to check for any signs of dysfunction in your brain stem. As long as no other complications arise, you'll be discharged home within the next 2 to 4 days. It could be a case of dizziness or vomiting that could prolong your hospitalization period. Symptoms like pain due to the incision and muscle spasms are common and can be relieved with medications. You should make sure to avoid heavy lifting or any other type of strenuous activities during the first few weeks after surgery. If your neurological functions had no problems before the operation, you'll be completely recovered within a month or two after the procedure. However, if you had any major neurological deficits before the surgery, you'll most likely require rehabilitation.

Follow up and consultation sessions will be required after the surgery. During these sessions, your doctor will ask you about the improvement or the persistence of your symptoms. In addition, he or she will inspect the incision area and will monitor the correct flow of the cerebrospinal fluid. If you had syringomyelia (a cyst filled with cerebrospinal fluid that forms in the central canal of the spinal cord) prior to the surgery, your doctor may ask for an MRI to confirm that the cyst responded correctly to the decompression. If you continue to have residual symptoms after the surgery such as neck pain or headache, your doctor will discuss with you the available options to determine the best treatment method for your case.

You should carefully weigh the pros and cons of the procedures prior to deciding to undergo another surgery. Although it's true that many patients experience some type of improvement after an operation, there's no guarantee that surgery will help every single patient. Keep in mind that the surgical procedures involved in the treatment of Chiari Malformation are rather complex. As a result, more than one surgery may be required to treat the condition. It is also important to remember that all surgeries carry risks. The most common complication observed in decompression surgery is the leakage of cerebrospinal fluid. The early detection and treatment of this outflow will prevent more serious complications. In addition, some other problems that may arise as a result of the surgery include reactions to anesthesia, bleeding, and infections. In a few cases, damage of the nerves, vertebra, brain stem, or spinal cord produced during the process of the surgery have led to the loss of mental functions, permanent brain damage, and other neurological deficits. Before deciding to receive surgery, you may want to consider consulting with an experienced neurosurgeon. It's also recommended that you see more than one specialist.

Seven: Research & Studies

Research and studies are constantly being performed to find more information about this condition. In particular, studies are being carried out regarding the genetic pathology of Chiari Malformation. Although a genetic prevalence was identified in some families, the exact genetic origin of this condition still remains unknown. Therefore, scientists keep working to discover the genes that may be responsible for causing the malformation by examining patients who have another family member with the malformation.

Studies and findings that have been made on the subject of Chiari Malformation include the following:

Studies have been conducted to evaluate the benefits of early surgical treatment in children. One particular study aimed to measure the benefits in children younger than 6 who had type I Chiari Malformation. In order to conduct the study, its authors identified 39 patients who had been diagnosed with this type of malformation before turning 6 and who had undergone surgery. After carefully analyzing their medical records, it was observed that almost 80% of the children between the ages of 0 and 2 presented oropharyngeal dysfunction (difficulties chewing and swallowing). Out of the children between the ages of 3 and 5, about 86% presented a cerebrospinal fluid cyst (syringomyelia) in the central canal of the spinal cord), 38% of them showed scoliosis (a sideways bent spine), and 57% suffered from headaches. All the patients went through surgery, and in most cases, the surgery had led to the resolution of the malformation or to the dramatic improvement of the initial symptoms. The study concluded that the early recognition of the disease together with the proper surgical treatment of type I Chiari Malformation in children leads to good outcomes in most patients.

Additional studies have been performed in order to determine whether early decompression of Chiari malformation in patients who also suffer from cerebrospinal fluid filled cysts (syringomyelia) resulted in stabilization or improvement of the associated scoliosis (lateral bending of the spine). The studies were based on the fact that Chiari I Malformation is often associated with scoliosis, particularly in the case of infant patients. Past data showed that the incidence of scoliosis in patients with Chiari malformation and syringomyelia was higher in the infant population. About 82% of patients younger than 20 years with syringomyelia presented scoliosis, while only 16% of patients older than 20 years showed this condition. Scoliasis in children can occur at very young ages and can progress very quickly. This particular study consisted of a twenty year review of surgical and nonsurgical treatment in a group of patients with Chiari Malformation who had also suffered from severe scoliosis. All of these patients had gone through decompression before turning 8. The research demonstrated that scoliosis can improve dramatically after the decompression of Chiari I Malformation and that early decompression of type I Chiari Malformation with syringomyelia and scoliosis resulted in improvement or stabilization of the spinal deformity. This eventually saved the patients from the need for spinal fusion, a surgical procedure that combines two or more vertebrae.

Post-surgery effects have also been the subject of analysis. A retrospective review of 192 patients who had undergone posterior fossa decompression showed that 36 of these 192 patients hadn't shown any improvement during a follow up period of up to 6 years after having gone through surgical decompression. An interesting point was that a large percentage of the patients who showed post-operative symptoms had presented coexisting type I Chiari Malformation and Pseudo-Tumor Cerebri (PTC), high cerebrospinal fluid pressure in the head, with no apparent cause. The symptoms of these patients varied, but most of them presented head pain of some sort. The studies showed that the surgical intervention itself could have caused changes in the flow of cerebrospinal fluid, which in turn could lead to the development of PTC after the surgery. So, it was concluded that in the cases of decompression surgery involving complications caused by increased intracranial pressure, additional procedures involving the drainage of cerebrospinal fluid should be taken into consideration. In addition, it was demonstrated that evaluating patients for high cerebrospinal fluid pressure before decompression surgery can also be of great value in assessing the chances of a positive surgical outcome.

Research has been performed regarding the possibility of less invasive treatment procedures since the current methods that are currently available involve complex, invasive surgeries. In 2009, a 15 year old boy with type I Chiari Malformation underwent a new, minimally invasive spine surgery procedure that was performed through his nose. The boy had come into the medical center presenting headaches, weakness in the arms, and difficulty in swallowing . Moreover, his speech was altered, and he was lacking his gag reflex. Once he was diagnosed with type I Chiari Malformation, the surgeons proceeded to remove a piece of bone from the back of his head to take pressure off of his brain stem. In order to do so in a less invasive way, the surgeons utilized a trans-nasal approach to get to his spinal cord. An endoscope with a light guide and a very small camera is used and surgical tools can be inserted to do a much less traumatic version of the original surgical procedure. The patient had a good recovery, and a month after the surgery, the symptoms were gone. Although this less invasive procedure had been used in adults in the past, this was the first time that it had been successfully performed on a child. This case showed that this procedure can be a viable alternative for children who suffer this type of malformation. Based on such results, the authors of the research strongly suggest magnetic resonance imaging in all patients with juvenile scoliosis when treatment options like spinal fusion are being considered, especially if it's the case of rapidly progressing scoliosis.

Eight: Brain Structure

No book about the brain would be complete without an overview of its anatomical parts and functions. In fact, knowing to the different parts of your brain—all of which perform different functions—can help alleviate fears when you have an illness or disease that affects a certain part of the brain.

The central nervous system is made up of your brain and spinal cord making it the center of your body's decision making and communications abilities. Together with the peripheral nervous system, the central nervous system controls every aspect of living and breathing, from tapping your fingers to memorizing the notes of a song.

Your nerves act as sensors, gathering information from your environment and sending that information to your brain, via your spinal cord. Your brain then interprets the message and sends a response to the rest of your body via the motor neurons.

Your brain is made of three major areas: the forebrain, midbrain, and hindbrain. The forebrain is broken up into the cerebrum, thalamus, and hypothalamus—which is part of the limbic system. In the midbrain you'll find the tectum and tegmentum and in the hindbrain there is the cerebellum, pons and medulla. The midbrain, pons, and medulla are often called the brainstem.

The largest part of your brain is the cerebrum or cortex, part of the forebrain. This is the part of the brain that controls thoughts and actions. The cerebrum is broken into four separate areas, or lobes: the frontal lobe, occipital lobe, parietal lobe, and temporal lobe. :

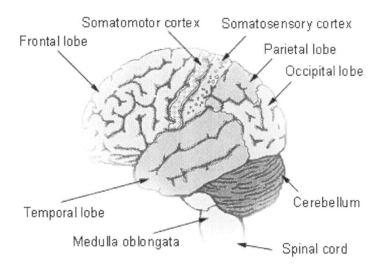

Lobes of the cerebrum

The frontal lobe controls emotions, movement, planning, problem solving, reasoning, and speech parts. The parietal lobe is also associated with movement, but it also controls movement, orientation, recognition, and stimuli perception. The occipital lobe is where all of the visual processing takes place and the temporal lobe controls auditory stimuli, memory, and speech.

The cerebrum is divided into two halves called the left and right hemispheres. They look almost the same, but there are slight differences in physical structure. The functions of the left hemisphere of the brain are verbal, rational, realistic, and rigid. Some problematic characteristics, which exist in the right hemisphere of the brain, are emotional comprehension and procession of symbols. The corpus callosum connects the two hemispheres. The cerebrum is made up of bundles of white nerve fibers, which carry signals to other parts of the body and your brain. These white nerve fibers are coated by a gray surface which is about a half inch thick.

The neocortex is a six-layered part of the cerebrum. The neocortex is the largest part of the cerebrum and is only found in mammals. Scientists think that the neocortex is a very recent part of the brain in terms of evolution and it is associated with higher brain functions and information processing.

The cerebellum is also divided into two hemispheres. The cerebellum is responsible for coordination and regulation of balance, posture, and movement.

Two hemispheres of the brain, from above

The limbic system, often called the "emotional brain", is buried inside the cerebrum. The limbic system contains the amygdala, hippocampus, hypothalamus, and thalamus.

The Limbic System

The amygdala, two almond shape groups of nuclei, have a primary role in processing of emotional reactions.

Amygdala

The hippocampus plays a primary role in long term memory and spatial navigation. The hypothalamus performs a variety of functions, including linking the endocrine system to the nervous system via the pituitary gland. The thalamus relays sensation, motor skills, and spatial sense to the cerebral cortex. The thalamus also has a primary role in sleep and consciousness.

The brain stem lies under the limbic system. The structure is responsible for vital life functions like breathing, heartbeat, sleep-wake cycle, consciousness and blood pressure.

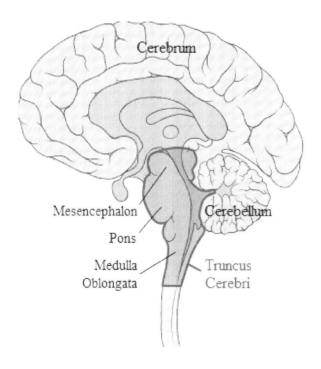

The brain stem (truncus cerebri) is made up of three parts: the midbrain, or mesencephalon, which is involved in vision, hearing, eye movement and body movement; the pons is a messenger and controls arousal and respiration; the medulla oblongata which controls heart rate and breathing rate.

Nine: Tests

Magnetic resonance imaging (MRI)

Magnetic resonance imaging is a painless and noninvasive method that uses radio waves to take a detailed three dimensional picture of the internal body parts. It provides an accurate view of your brain, cerebellum, and spinal cord. An MRI will show whether you have an excessive build up of cerebrospinal fluid and whether there's been any loss of brain tissue. In addition, it will provide information on the extent of any malformations, and it'll serve to give an idea of your disease's progression. However, MRIs are not as effective in showing bone related injuries. X-rays will be used for that.

For an MRI, you'll likely be dressed in a paper thin hospital gown and guided into a tunnel-like tube. Depending on how complex your case is, you could be inside the machine for an hour. The machine is loud, so you may be given sound canceling headphones or earplugs. Some patients experience claustrophobia inside the MRI, so make sure you talk to your doctor about the possibility of a sedative if you don't like confined spaces.

MRI Machine

MRI doesn't involve ionizing radiation, like X-rays and CT scans. MRI uses the water inside your body to produce an image. The MRI provides superior, high resolution images and can also provide chemical information about your brain as well. The procedure is safe and commonplace: tens of millions of scans are performed every year. An MRI is the diagnostic tool of choice for soft tissue like the brain and spinal column.

The MRI is actually a massive magnet that weighs tens of thousands of pounds and is capable of creating a magnetic field. It's for that reason you won't be allowed to take any metal objects into the room: they can become life threatening projectiles. You won't be allowed to have an MRI if you are fitted with a pacemaker or an aneurism clip. You might not be able to have an MRI if you have any shrapnel in your body. The ink in tattoos could heat up, although this is rarely a problem. Tooth fillings and braces might cause an itching sensation and they may cause a disturbance to images of the brain, so make sure you talk with your physician or technologist about this possibility.

You may be injected with a contrast dye called gadolinium, which will make some images clearer. Once you're inside the MRI, the technologist will talk to you from the control room. Your head will be in the center of the machine. The water in your body is made up from a large number of oxygen and hydrogen atoms. The hydrogen atom has a nucleus with a positively charged proton that spins on a randomly oriented axis. When the MRI is turned on, most of the hydrogen atoms line up along the magnetic field. Some will not, and it's those hydrogen atoms that the MRI "reads" to produce your image. The protons absorb a radio frequency pulse and flip back and forth when the radio frequency is turned on and off. This emits a signal to the radio frequency coil, which is turned into an electric current and then a digital image.

MRI scans display more than 250 shades of grey, which show variations in tissue density or water content.

MRI of a normal brain

MRI Showing a Chiari Malformation

X-rays

X-rays: In most cases, an X-ray of your head and your neck will be taken in addition to an MRI. X-rays are safe and painless, and they'll produce an image of the bones and some of the tissues on film. Even though an X-ray by itself cannot reveal malformations in the brain, it can still be useful to show any bone abnormalities that are often associated with this condition. Radiographs are produced with a variety of imaging tools which all require exposing you to some amount of X-ray radiation. The image is a shadow of those parts of your body that block or absorb the radiation; it's actually a negative of your body—dark parts on the image are white areas on your body that blocked the X-rays. The image is collected on a digital imaging plate, on a photosensitive film, or it can be seen on a special kind of screen by your physician.

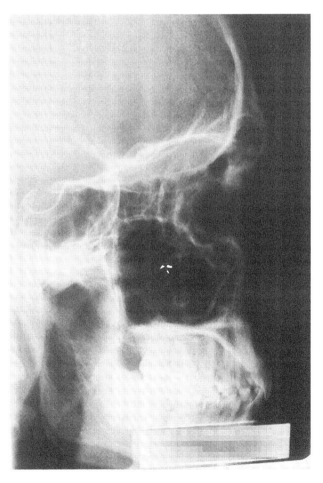

Head X-Ray

Computed tomography (CT scan)

Computed tomography (CT scan): This painless and non-invasive method produces two-dimensional pictures of the bones, vascular irregularities, certain brain tumors and cysts using X-rays. Therefore, it can show the existence of any brain damage or any other disorders. In addition, CT scans will serve to check whether you have any of the bone abnormalities associated with CM or hydrocephalus and/or whether you have an excessive buildup of cerebrospinal fluid. Keep in mind that CT scans are less effective for analyzing your spinal cord.

Like the MRI, the CT scan may also be performed with the aid of a contrast agent, injected just before the procedure starts. The images produced by a CT scan are called sections, or cuts, because they look like cross sections of your brain.

Brain stem auditory evoked Response (BAER)

Brain stem auditory evoked response(BAER)/ Brainstem Evoked response Audiometry (BERA): This is an electrical screening test that helps to examine the correct functioning of your hearing apparatus and your brain stem connections. This test will be useful in determining whether your brainstem is functioning properly.

The hearing test detects electrical activity in the auditory pathways in your brain in much the same way that an antenna might detect a TV signal. The BAER produces a graph with a series of peaks and troughs: a flat line indicates deafness.

In order to collect the signals, you'll have a number of small electrodes placed on your scalp and ears. You'll lie down on a chair or flat surface and listen to a series of clicks for about 15-30 minutes.

Myleogram: A myelogram is a type of x-ray where a contrast material is injected into the fluid-filled space around your spinal cord to detect any pathology including the location of a spinal cord injury, cysts, and tumors. . You'll lie on your side or stomach on an X-ray table and you'll be given local anesthetic. A needle will be inserted into your spinal canal and an oil or water based contrast will be injected. After the X-rays, you'll have to remain lying in bed for 24 hours after the procedure. For this process, you'll be first inserted a contrast material into your cerebrospinal fluid space. Then, an X-ray of the spinal cord will be taken to check its pressure. Although this method was frequently used in the past, its usage has greatly decreased now.

Somatosensory Evoked Potentials (SSEP): This is an electrical test of the nerves that are involved in sensation. The results of the test provide information about the spinal cord and the functioning of the brain. Electrodes will be placed on your scalp and your physician will look for the size and height of the peaks.

Ten: What to Expect from Brain Surgery

No matter what advances have been made in modern medicine, brain surgery is a frightening experience for anyone. Your brain is the center of who you are, and when you're facing brain surgery the prospect of someone cutting your core can be the ultimate violation. When you visit the neurosurgeon, don't visit them alone: take a trusted friend or relative with you so that they can remember all of the things you probably won't.

Tests

You'll likely have a series of tests to check your overall health before your surgery. These tests might include an electroencephalograph (EEG) which records your brain waves or an angiogram to show the placement of your blood vessels so that your surgeon can avoid them. You will likely have a series of tests called neurological exam, where an examining physician will ask you to squeeze his hand or to pull your legs up at a certain height . These tests give your physicians a baseline of your neurological status before your surgery. You might also have blood tests, lung X-rays, or an echocardiogram (ECG).

Important questions to ask your neurosurgeon before your scheduled surgery:

What is the success rate of the surgical procedure?

How many of my particular type of surgeries have you performed?

What is the length of my procedure?

What exactly are you going to do during the procedure?

What is my recovery time?

How long will I be in the hospital?

Are there any expected side effects or potential complications?

Will you be using staples or absorbable stitches?

What type of incision will I have and where will it be?

Will my head be shaved?

There are two major types of brain surgery:

Craniotomy and Endonasal surgery.

A craniotomy involves making an incision in your skull to access the part of your brain requiring surgery. Some areas at the base of the brain can be accessed through the nasal cavity and sinuses, which means a surgeon can perform endonasal/transnasal surgery .

After craniotomy:

You'll likely spend a day in the intensive care unit (ICU) and at least two nights on a regular ward. You might be given a CT scan or MRI before you are discharged.

For the first week after your surgery, avoid heavy lifting, straining, and bending over. Don't drive or exercise for at least two weeks after your surgery, although you can walk.

After endonasal surgery

You'll likely spend two nights in the hospital in a regular ward.

Most patients will spend two nights on a regular (non-ICU) ward and you may have a CT scan or MRI before you are discharged from the hospital.

Common after effects of brain surgery

Headaches -

Headaches after brain surgery are very common and are a result of injury to the brain. Depending on the extent of your surgery, you could suffer from headaches for years afterwards.

Nasal bleeding and discharge

If you had endonasal surgery, nasal discharge and stuffiness are common.

Itching -

It's very likely that you will experience itching and discomfort along the incision site. You may also hear a clicking where the bone plates rub together.

Medications -

Anticonvulsants: You will probably be on an anticonvulsant medication to control or prevent seizures caused by brain trauma.

Steroids: you may be given steroids to reduce swelling, and other inflammatory signs and symptoms which are common after any kind of surgery.

    Fatigue -

Fatigue is very common after brain surgery. You'll likely feel weak throughout the first few weeks after surgery. Fatigue can be persistent and may last for many months.

    Short term memory loss

    Many people experience a momentary amnesia, especially short term memory loss, after brain surgery.

    Depression, fear, and anger

    Depression, fear and anger are typical stages a patient goes through after a brain surgery, especially if the procedure was unexpected.

    Numbness at the incision site -

This is a very common side effect of surgery and is completely normal.

Dizziness

You may feel dizzy after your surgery. This is a very common complaint for post surgical patients.

Chest Infections

Breathing exercises will help you to avoid a chest infection after surgery, which can happen if you are not able to move around as much as you normally can.

Blood Clots

Blood clots can occur after surgery if you are immobile for a long time. Leg exercises can stop these clots from forming.

Transfer to a rehabilitation center -

You may be transferred to a rehabilitation center after your surgery. An army of professionals including physical therapists, occupational therapists, and speech therapists, will work with you to overcome any functional problems after your surgery.

When To Call The Doctor:

Call your physician if you have any of the following signs or symptoms following your surgery:

Fever

Clear, watery Drainage from the incisions or bloody leaks

redness and swelling around incision area

Seizures

Sudden severe headache or persistent headache not relived by rest and medication

Stiff Neck, nausea, vomiting, or diarrhea

New vision problems like blurring or double vision

Eleven: A Genetics Primer

Although genetics can't cure any disease, understanding how and why genetic defects occur can help stop the gene from transmitting from parent to child.

Genetics (from Ancient Greek γενετικός genetikos, "genitive" and that from γένεσις genesis, "origin"[1][2][3]), a discipline of biology, is the science of genes, heredity, and variation in living organisms.[4][5] The fact that living things inherit traits from their parents has been used since prehistoric times to improve crop plants and animals through selective breeding. However, the modern science of genetics, which seeks to understand the process of inheritance, only began with the work of Gregor Mendel in the mid-19th century.[6] Although he did not know the physical basis for heredity, Mendel observed that organisms inherit traits via discrete units of inheritance, which are now called genes.

Genes correspond to regions within DNA, a molecule composed of a chain of four different types of nucleotides—the sequence of these nucleotides is the genetic information organisms inherit. DNA naturally occurs in a double stranded form, with nucleotides on each strand complementary to each other. Each strand can act as a template for creating a new partner strand—this is the physical method for making copies of genes that can be inherited.

The sequence of nucleotides in a gene is translated by cells to produce a chain of amino acids, creating proteins—the order of amino acids in a protein corresponds to the order of nucleotides in the gene. This relationship between nucleotide sequence and amino acid sequence is known as the genetic code. The amino acids in a protein determine how it folds into a three-dimensional shape; this structure is, in turn, responsible for the protein's function. Proteins carry out almost all the functions needed for cells to live. A change to the DNA in a gene can change a protein's amino acids, changing its shape and function: this can have a dramatic effect in the cell and on the organism as a whole.

Although genetics plays a large role in the appearance and behavior of organisms, it is the combination of genetics with what an organism experiences that determines the ultimate outcome. For example, while genes play a role in determining an organism's size, the nutrition and other conditions it experiences after inception also have a large effect.

History of genetics

DNA, the molecular basis for inheritance. Each strand of DNA is a chain of nucleotides, matching each other in the center to form what look like rungs on a twisted ladder.

Although the science of genetics began with the applied and theoretical work of Gregor Mendel in the mid-19th century, other theories of inheritance preceded Mendel. A popular theory during Mendel's time was the concept of blending inheritance: the idea that individuals inherit a smooth blend of traits from their parents. Mendel's work disproved this, showing that traits are composed of combinations of distinct genes rather than a continuous blend. Another theory that had some support at that time was the inheritance of acquired characteristics: the belief that individuals inherit traits strengthened by their parents. This theory (commonly associated with Jean-Baptiste Lamarck) is now known to be wrong—the experiences of individuals do not affect the genes they pass to their children.[7] Other theories included the pangenesis of Charles Darwin (which had both acquired and inherited aspects) and Francis Galton's reformulation of pangenesis as both particulate and inherited.[8]

Mendelian and classical genetics

The modern science of genetics traces its roots to Gregor Johann Mendel, a German-Czech Augustinian monk and scientist who studied the nature of inheritance in plants. In his paper "Versuche über Pflanzenhybriden" ("Experiments on Plant Hybridization"), presented in 1865 to the Natur forschender Verein (Society for Research in Nature) in Brünn, Mendel traced the inheritance patterns of certain traits in pea plants and described them mathematically.[9] Although this pattern of inheritance could only be observed for a few traits, Mendel's work suggested that heredity was particulate, not acquired, and that the inheritance patterns of many traits could be explained through simple rules and ratios.

The importance of Mendel's work did not gain wide understanding until the 1890s, after his death, when other scientists working on similar problems re-discovered his research. William Bateson, a proponent of Mendel's work, coined the word genetics in 1905.[10][11] (The adjective genetic, derived from the Greek word genesis—γένεσις, "origin" and that from the word genno—γεννώ, "to give birth", predates the noun and was first used in a biological sense in 1860.)[12] Bateson popularized the usage of the word genetics to describe the study of inheritance in his inaugural address to the Third International Conference on Plant Hybridization in London, England, in 1906.[13]

After the rediscovery of Mendel's work, scientists tried to determine which molecules in the cell were responsible for inheritance. In 1910, Thomas Hunt Morgan argued that genes are on chromosomes, based on observations of a sex-linked white eye mutation in fruit flies.[14] In 1913, his student Alfred Sturtevant used the phenomenon of genetic linkage to show that genes are arranged linearly on the chromosome.[15]

Morgan's observation of sex-linked inheritance of a mutation causing white eyes in Drosophila led him to the hypothesis that genes are located upon chromosomes.

[Molecular genetics

Although genes were known to exist on chromosomes, chromosomes are composed of both protein and DNA—scientists did not know which of these is responsible for inheritance. In 1928, Frederick Griffith discovered the phenomenon of transformation (see Griffith's experiment): dead bacteria could transfer genetic material to "transform" other still-living bacteria. Sixteen years later, in 1944, Oswald Theodore Avery, Colin McLeod and Maclyn McCarty identified the molecule responsible for transformation as DNA.[16] The Hershey-Chase experiment in 1952 also showed that DNA (rather than protein) is the genetic material of the viruses that infect bacteria, providing further evidence that DNA is the molecule responsible for inheritance.[17]

James D. Watson and Francis Crick determined the structure of DNA in 1953, using the X-ray crystallography work of Rosalind Franklin and Maurice Wilkins that indicated DNA had a helical structure (i.e., shaped like a corkscrew).[18][19] Their double-helix model had two strands of DNA with the nucleotides pointing inward, each matching a complementary nucleotide on the other strand to form what looks like rungs on a twisted ladder.[20] This structure showed that genetic information exists in the sequence of nucleotides on each strand of DNA. The structure also suggested a simple method for duplication: if the strands are separated, new partner strands can be reconstructed for each based on the sequence of the old strand.

Although the structure of DNA showed how inheritance works, it was still not known how DNA influences the behavior of cells. In the following years, scientists tried to understand how DNA controls the process of protein production. It was discovered that the cell uses DNA as a template to create matching messenger RNA (a molecule with nucleotides, very similar to DNA). The nucleotide sequence of a messenger RNA is used to create an amino acid sequence in protein; this translation between nucleotide and amino acid sequences is known as the genetic code.

With this molecular understanding of inheritance, an explosion of research became possible. One important development was chain-termination DNA sequencing in 1977 by Frederick Sanger. This technology allows scientists to read the nucleotide sequence of a DNA molecule.[21] In 1983, Kary Banks Mullis developed the polymerase chain reaction, providing a quick way to isolate and amplify a specific section of a DNA from a mixture.[22] Through the pooled efforts of the Human Genome Project and the parallel private effort by

Celera Genomics, these and other techniques culminated in the sequencing of the human genome in 2003.[23]

Mendelian inheritance

At its most fundamental level, inheritance in organisms occurs by means of discrete traits, called genes.[24] This property was first observed by Gregor Mendel, who studied the segregation of heritable traits in pea plants.[9][25] In his experiments studying the trait for flower color, Mendel observed that the flowers of each pea plant were either purple or white—but never an intermediate between the two colors. These different, discrete versions of the same gene are called alleles.

In the case of pea, which is a diploid species, each individual plant has two alleles of each gene, one allele inherited from each parent.[26] Many species, including humans, have this pattern of inheritance. Diploid organisms with two copies of the same allele of a given gene are called homozygous at that gene locus, while organisms with two different alleles of a given gene are called heterozygous.

The set of alleles for a given organism is called its genotype, while the observable traits of the organism are called its phenotype. When organisms are heterozygous at a gene, often one allele is called dominant as its qualities dominate the phenotype of the organism, while the other allele is called recessive as its qualities recede and are not observed. Some alleles do not have complete dominance and instead have incomplete dominance by expressing an intermediate phenotype, or codominance by expressing both alleles at once.[27]

When a pair of organisms reproduce sexually, their offspring randomly inherit one of the two alleles from each parent. These observations of discrete inheritance and the segregation of alleles are collectively known as Mendel's first law or the Law of Segregation.

Geneticists use diagrams and symbols to describe inheritance. A gene is represented by one or a few letters. Often a "+" symbol is used to mark the usual, non-mutant allele for a gene.[28]

In fertilization and breeding experiments (and especially when discussing Mendel's laws) the parents are referred to as the "P" generation and the offspring as the "F1" (first filial) generation. When the F1 offspring mate with each other, the offspring are called the "F2" (second filial) generation. One of the common diagrams used to predict the result of cross-breeding is the Punnett square.

When studying human genetic diseases, geneticists often use pedigree chartsto represent the inheritance of traits.[29] These charts map the inheritance of a trait in a family tree.

Interactions of multiple genes

Human height is a complex genetic trait. Francis Galton's data from 1889 shows the relationship between offspring height as a function of mean parent height. While correlated, remaining variation in offspring heights indicates environment is also an important factor in this trait.

Organisms have thousands of genes, and in sexually reproducing organisms these genes generally assort independently of each other. This means that the inheritance of an allele for yellow or green pea color is unrelated to the inheritance of alleles for white or purple flowers. This phenomenon, known as "Mendel's second law" or the "Law of independent assortment", means that the alleles of different genes get shuffled between parents to form offspring with many different combinations. (Some genes do not assort independently, demonstrating genetic linkage, a topic discussed later in this chapter.)

Often different genes can interact in a way that influences the same trait. In the Blue-eyed Mary (Omphalodes verna), for example, there exists a gene with alleles that determine the color of flowers: blue or magenta. Another gene, however, controls whether the flowers have color at all or are white. When a plant has two copies of this white allele, its flowers are white—regardless of whether the first gene has blue or magenta alleles. This interaction between genes is called epistasis, with the second gene epistatic to the first.[30]

Many traits are not discrete features (e.g. purple or white flowers) but are instead continuous features (e.g. human height and skin color). These complex traits are products of many genes.[31] The influence of these genes is mediated, to varying degrees, by the environment an organism has experienced. The degree to which an organism's genes contribute to a complex trait is called heritability.[32] Measurement of the heritability of a trait is relative—in a more variable environment, the environment has a bigger influence on the total variation of the trait. For example, human height is a complex trait with a heritability of 89% in the United States. In Nigeria, however, where people experience a more variable access to good nutrition and health care, height has a heritability of only 62%.[33]

DNA and Chromosome

The molecular structure of DNA. Bases pair through the arrangement of hydrogen bonding between the strands.

The molecular basis for genes is deoxyribonucleic acid (DNA). DNA is composed of a chain of nucleotides, of which there are four types: adenine (A), cytosine (C),guanine (G), and thymine (T). Genetic information exists in the sequence of these nucleotides, and genes exist as stretches of sequence along the DNA chain.[34]Viruses are the only exception to this rule—sometimes viruses use the very similar molecule RNA instead of DNA as their genetic material.[35]

DNA normally exists as a double-stranded molecule, coiled into the shape of a double-helix. Each nucleotide in DNA preferentially pairs with its partner nucleotide on the opposite strand: A pairs with T, and C pairs with G. Thus, in its two-stranded form, each strand effectively contains all necessary information, redundant with its partner strand. This structure of DNA is the physical basis for inheritance: DNA replication duplicates the genetic information by splitting the strands and using each strand as a template for synthesis of a new partner strand.[36]

Genes are arranged linearly along long chains of DNA sequence, called chromosomes. In bacteria, each cell usually contains a single circular chromosome, while eukaryotic organisms (including plants and animals) have their DNA arranged in multiple linear chromosomes. These DNA strands are often extremely long; the largest human chromosome, for example, is about 247 million base pairs in length.[37] The DNA of a chromosome is associated with structural proteins that organize, compact, and control access to the DNA, forming a material called chromatin; in eukaryotes, chromatin is usually composed of nucleosomes, segments of DNA wound around cores of histone proteins.[38] The full set of hereditary material in an organism (usually the combined DNA sequences of all chromosomes) is called the genome.

While haploid organisms have only one copy of each chromosome, most animals and many plants are diploid, containing two of each chromosome and thus two copies of every gene.[26] The two alleles for a gene are located on identical loci of sister chromatids, each allele inherited from a different parent.

Walther Flemming's 1882 diagram of eukaryotic cell division. Chromosomes are copied, condensed, and organized. Then, as the cell divides, chromosome copies separate into the daughter cells.

An exception exists in the sex chromosomes, specialized chromosomes many animals have evolved that play a role in determining the sex of an organism.[39] In humans and other mammals, the Y chromosome has very few genes and triggers the development of male sexual characteristics, while the X chromosome is similar to the other chromosomes and contains many genes unrelated to sex determination. Females have two copies of the X chromosome, but males have one Y and only one X chromosome; this difference in X chromosome copy numbers leads to the unusual inheritance patterns of sex-linked disorders.

Asexual reproduction and Sexual reproduction

When cells divide, their full genome is copied and each daughter cell inherits one copy. This process, called mitosis, is the simplest form of reproduction and is the basis for asexual reproduction. Asexual reproduction can also occur in multicellular organisms, producing offspring that inherit their genome from a single parent. Offspring that are genetically identical to their parents are called clones.

Eukaryotic organisms often use sexual reproduction to generate offspring that contain a mixture of genetic material inherited from two different parents. The process of sexual reproduction alternates between forms that contain single copies of the genome (haploid) and double copies (diploid).[26] Haploid cells fuse and combine genetic material to create a diploid cell with paired chromosomes. Diploid organisms form haploids by dividing, without replicating their DNA, to create daughter cells that randomly inherit one of each pair of chromosomes. Most animals and many plants are diploid for most of their lifespan, with the haploid form reduced to single cell gametes such as sperm or eggs.

Although they do not use the haploid/diploid method of sexual reproduction, bacteria have many methods of acquiring new genetic information. Some bacteria can undergo conjugation, transferring a small circular piece of DNA to another bacterium.[40] Bacteria can also take up raw DNA fragments found in the environment and integrate them into their genomes, a phenomenon known as transformation.[41] These processes result in horizontal gene transfer, transmitting fragments of genetic information between organisms that would be otherwise unrelated.

Chromosomal crossover and Genetic linkage

Thomas Hunt Morgan's 1916 illustration of a double crossover between chromosomes

The diploid nature of chromosomes allows for genes on different chromosomes to assort independently during sexual reproduction, recombining to form new combinations of genes. Genes on the same chromosome would theoretically never recombine, however, were it not for the process of chromosomal crossover. During crossover, chromosomes exchange stretches of DNA, effectively shuffling the gene alleles between the chromosomes.[42] This process of chromosomal crossover generally occurs during meiosis, a series of cell divisions that creates haploid cells.

The probability of chromosomal crossover occurring between two given points on the chromosome is related to the distance between the points. For an arbitrarily long distance, the probability of crossover is high enough that the inheritance of the genes is effectively uncorrelated. For genes that are closer together, however, the lower probability of crossover means that the genes demonstrate genetic linkage—alleles for the two genes tend to be inherited together. The amounts of linkage between a series of genes can be combined to form a linear linkage map that roughly describes the arrangement of the genes along the chromosome.[43]

Genetic code

Genes generally express their functional effect through the production of proteins, which are complex molecules responsible for most functions in the cell. Proteins are chains of amino acids, and the DNA sequence of a gene (through an RNA intermediate) is used to produce a specific protein sequence. This process begins with the production of an RNA molecule with a sequence matching the gene's DNA sequence, a process called transcription.

This messenger RNA molecule is then used to produce a corresponding amino acid sequence through a process called translation. Each group of three nucleotides in the sequence, called a codon, corresponds to one of the twenty possible amino acids in protein; this correspondence is called the genetic code.[44] The flow of information is unidirectional: information is transferred from nucleotide sequences into the amino acid sequence of proteins, but it never transfers from protein back into the sequence of DNA—a phenomenon Francis Crick called the central dogma of molecular biology.[45]

The specific sequence of amino acids results in a unique three-dimensional structure for that protein, and the three-dimensional structures of proteins are related to their functions.[46][47] Some are simple structural molecules, like the fibers formed by the protein collagen. Proteins can bind to other proteins and simple molecules, sometimes acting as enzymes by facilitating chemical reactions within the bound molecules (without changing the structure of the protein itself). Protein structure is dynamic; the protein hemoglobin bends into slightly different forms as it facilitates the capture, transport, and release of oxygen molecules within mammalian blood.

The dynamic structure of hemoglobin is responsible for its ability to transport oxygen within mammalian blood.

A single nucleotide difference within DNA can cause a change in the amino acid sequence of a protein. Because protein structures are the result of their amino acid sequences, some changes can dramatically change the properties of a protein by destabilizing the structure or changing the surface of the protein in a way that changes its interaction with other proteins and molecules. For example, sickle-cell anemia is a human genetic disease that results from a single base difference within the coding region for the βglobin section of hemoglobin, causing a single amino acid change that changes hemoglobin's physical properties.[48] Sickle-cell versions of hemoglobin stick to themselves, stacking to form fibers that distort the shape of red blood cells carrying the protein. These sickle-shaped cells no longer flow smoothly through blood vessels, having a tendency to clog or degrade, causing the medical problems associated with this disease.

Some genes are transcribed into RNA but are not translated into protein products—such RNA molecules are called non-coding RNA. In some cases, these products fold into structures which are involved in critical cell functions (e.g. ribosomal RNA and transfer RNA). RNA can also have regulatory effect through hybridization interactions with other RNA molecules (e.g. microRNA).

Nature versus nurture

Although genes contain all the information an organism uses to function, the environment plays an important role in determining the ultimate phenotype—a phenomenon often referred to as "nature vs. nurture". The phenotype of an organism depends on the interaction of genetics with the environment. One example of this is the case of temperature-sensitive mutations. Often, a single amino acid change within the sequence of a protein does not change its behavior and interactions with other molecules, but it does destabilize the structure. In a high temperature environment, where molecules are moving more quickly and hitting each other, this results in the protein losing its structure and failing to function. In a low temperature environment, however, the protein's structure is stable and it functions normally. This type of mutation is visible in the coat coloration of Siamese cats, where a mutation in an enzyme responsible for pigment production causes it to destabilize and lose function at high temperatures.[49] The protein remains functional in areas of skin that are colder—legs, ears, tail, and face—and so the cat has dark fur at its extremities.

Environment also plays a dramatic role in effects of the human genetic disease phenylketonuria.[50] The mutation that causes phenylketonuria disrupts the ability of the body to break down the amino acid phenylalanine, causing a toxic build-up of an intermediate molecule that, in turn, causes severe symptoms of progressive mental retardation and seizures. If someone with the phenylketonuria mutation follows a strict diet that avoids this amino acid, however, they remain normal and healthy.

A popular method to determine how much role nature and nurture play is to study identical and fraternal twins or siblings of multiple birth.[citation needed]Because identical siblings come from the same zygote they are genetically the same. Fraternal siblings however are as different genetically from one another as normal siblings. By comparing how often the twin of a set has the same disorder between fraternal and identical twins, scientists can see whether there is more of a nature or nurture effect. One famous example of a multiple birth study includes the Genain quadruplets, who were identical quadruplets all diagnosed with schizophrenia.[51]

Regulation of gene expression

The genome of a given organism contains thousands of genes, but not all these genes need to be active at any given moment. A gene is expressed when it is being transcribed into mRNA (and translated into protein), and there exist many cellular methods of controlling the expression of genes such that proteins are produced only when needed by the cell. Transcription factors are regulatory proteins that bind to the start of genes, either promoting or inhibiting the transcription of the gene.[52] Within the genome of Escherichia coli bacteria, for example, there exists a series of genes necessary for the synthesis of the amino acid tryptophan. However, when tryptophan is already available to the cell, these genes for tryptophan synthesis are no longer needed. The presence of tryptophan directly affects the activity of the genes—tryptophan molecules bind to the tryptophan repressor (a transcription factor), changing the repressor's structure such that the repressor binds to the genes. The tryptophan repressor blocks the transcription and expression of the genes, thereby creating negative feedback regulation of the tryptophan synthesis process.[53]

Transcription factors bind to DNA, influencing the transcription of associated genes.

Differences in gene expression are especially clear within multi cellular organisms, where cells all contain the same genome but have very different structures and behaviors due to the expression of different sets of genes. All the cells in a multi cellular organism derive from a single cell, differentiating into variant cell types in response to external and intercellular signals and gradually establishing different patterns of gene expression to create different behaviors. As no single gene is responsible for the development of structures within multi cellular organisms, these patterns arise from the complex interactions between many cells.

Within eukaryotes there exist structural features of chromatin that influence the transcription of genes, often in the form of modifications to DNA and chromatin that are stably inherited by daughter cells.[54] These features are called "epigenetic" because they exist "on top" of the DNA sequence and retain inheritance from one cell generation to the next. Because of epigenetic features, different cell types grown within the same medium can retain very different properties. Although epigenetic features are generally dynamic over the course of development, some, like the phenomenon of paramutation, have multigenerational inheritance and exist as rare exceptions to the general rule of DNA as the basis for inheritance.[55]

Mutation

Gene duplication allows diversification by providing redundancy: one gene can mutate and lose its original function without harming the organism.

During the process of DNA replication, errors occasionally occur in the polymerization of the second strand. These errors, called mutations, can have an impact on the phenotype of an organism, especially if they occur within the protein coding sequence of a gene. Error rates are usually very low—1 error in every 10–100 million bases—due to the "proofreading" ability of DNA polymerases.[56][57] (Without proofreading error rates are a thousandfold higher; because many viruses rely on DNA and RNA polymerases that lack proofreading ability, they experience higher mutation rates.) Processes that increase the rate of changes in DNA are called mutagenic: mutagenic chemicals promote errors in DNA replication, often by interfering with the structure of base-pairing, while UV radiation induces mutations by causing damage to the DNA structure.[58]Chemical damage to DNA occurs naturally as well, and cells use DNA repair mechanisms to repair mismatches and breaks in DNA—nevertheless, the repair sometimes fails to return the DNA to its original sequence.

In organisms that use chromosomal crossover to exchange DNA and recombine genes, errors in alignment during meiosis can also cause mutations.[59] Errors in crossover are especially likely when similar sequences cause partner chromosomes to adopt a mistaken alignment; this makes some regions in genomes more prone to mutating in this way. These errors create large structural changes in DNA sequence—duplications, inversions or deletions of entire regions, or the accidental exchanging of whole parts between different chromosomes (called translocation).

Evolution

Mutations alter an organisms genotype and occasionally this causes different phenotypes to appear. Most mutations have little effect on an organism's phenotype, health, or reproductive fitness. Mutations that do have an effect are usually deleterious, but occasionally some can be beneficial. Studies in the fly Drosophila melanogaster suggest that if a mutation changes a protein produced by a gene, about 70 percent of these mutations will be harmful with the remainder being either neutral or weakly beneficial.[60]

Population genetics studies the distribution of genetic differences within populations and how these distributions change over time.[61]Changes in the frequency of an allele in a population are mainly influenced by natural selection, where a given allele provides a selective or reproductive advantage to the organism,[62] as well as other factors such as genetic drift, artificial selection and migration.[63]

Over many generations, the genomes of organisms can change significantly, resulting in the phenomenon of evolution. Selection for beneficial mutations can cause a species to evolve into forms better able to survive in their environment, a process called adaptation.[64] New species are formed through the process of speciation, often caused by geographical separations that prevent populations from exchanging genes with each other.[65] The application of genetic principles to the study of population biology and evolution is referred to as the modern synthesis.

By comparing the homology between different species' genomes it is possible to calculate the evolutionary distance between them and when they may have diverged (called a molecular clock).[66] Genetic comparisons are generally considered a more accurate method of characterizing the relatedness between species than the comparison of phenotypic characteristics.[citation needed] The evolutionary distances between species can be used to form evolutionary trees; these trees represent the common descent and divergence of species over time, although they do not show the transfer of genetic material between unrelated species (known as horizontal gene transfer and most common in bacteria).

Although geneticists originally studied inheritance in a wide range of organisms, researchers began to specialize in studying the genetics of a particular subset of organisms. The fact that significant research already existed for a given organism would encourage new researchers to choose it for further study, and so eventually a few model organisms became the basis for most genetics research.[67] Common research topics in model organism genetics include the study of gene regulationand the involvement of genes in development and cancer.

Organisms were chosen, in part, for convenience—short generation times and easy genetic manipulation made some organisms popular genetics research tools. Widely used model organisms include the gut bacterium Escherichia coli, the plant Arabidopsis thaliana, baker's yeast (Saccharomyces cerevisiae), the nematode Caenorhabditis elegans, the common fruit fly (Drosophila melanogaster), and the common house mouse (Mus musculus).

Medical genetics research

Medical genetics seeks to understand how genetic variation relates to human health and disease.[68] When searching for an unknown gene that may be involved in a disease, researchers commonly use genetic linkage and genetic pedigree charts to find the location on the genome associated with the disease. At the population level, researchers take advantage of Mendelian randomization to look for locations in the genome that are associated with diseases, a technique especially useful for multigenic traits not clearly defined by a single gene.[69] Once a candidate gene is found, further research is often done on the corresponding gene (called an orthologous gene) in model organisms. In addition to studying genetic diseases, the increased availability of genotyping techniques has led to the field of pharmacogenetics—studying how genotype can affect drug responses.[70]

Individuals differ in their inherited tendency to develop cancer,[71] and cancer is a genetic disease.[72] The process of cancer development in the body is a combination of events. Mutations occasionally occur within cells in the body as they divide. Although these mutations will not be inherited by any offspring, they can affect the behavior of cells, sometimes causing them to grow and divide more frequently. There are biological mechanisms that attempt to stop this process; signals are given to inappropriately dividing cells that should trigger cell death, but sometimes additional mutations occur that cause cells to ignore these messages. An internal process of natural selection occurs within the body and eventually mutations accumulate within cells to promote their own growth, creating a cancerous tumor that grows and invades various tissues of the body.

Research techniques

DNA can be manipulated in the laboratory. Restriction enzymes are commonly used enzymes that cut DNA at specific sequences, producing predictable fragments of DNA.[73] DNA fragments can be visualized through use of gel electrophoresis, which separates fragments according to their length.

The use of ligation enzymes allows DNA fragments to be connected, and by ligating fragments of DNA together from different sources, researchers can create recombinant DNA. Often associated with genetically modified organisms, recombinant DNA is commonly used in the context of plasmids—short circular DNA fragments with a few genes on them. By inserting plasmids into bacteria and growing those bacteria on plates of agar (to isolate clones of bacteria cells), researchers can clonally amplify the inserted fragment of DNA (a process known as molecular cloning). (Cloning can also refer to the creation of clonal organisms, through various techniques.)

DNA can also be amplified using a procedure called the polymerase chain reaction (PCR).[74] By using specific short sequences of DNA, PCR can isolate and exponentially amplify a targeted region of DNA. Because it can amplify from extremely small amounts of DNA, PCR is also often used to detect the presence of specific DNA sequences.

DNA sequencing and genomics

One of the most fundamental technologies developed to study genetics, DNA sequencing allows researchers to determine the sequence of nucleotides in DNA fragments. Developed in 1977 by Frederick Sanger and coworkers, chain-termination sequencing is now routinely used to sequence DNA fragments.[75] With this technology, researchers have been able to study the molecular sequences associated with many human diseases.

As sequencing has become less expensive, researchers have sequenced the genomes of many organisms, using computational tools to stitch together the sequences of many different fragments (a process called genome assembly).[76] These technologies were used to sequence the human genome, leading to the completion of the Human Genome Project in 2003.[23] New high-throughput sequencing technologies are dramatically lowering the cost of DNA sequencing, with many researchers hoping to bring the cost of resequencing a human genome down to a thousand dollars.[77]

The large amount of sequence data available has created the field of genomics, research that uses computational tools to search for and analyze patterns in the full genomes of organisms. Genomics can also be considered a subfield of bioinformatics, which uses computational approaches to analyze large sets of biological data.

Notes

1. Genetikos, Henry George Liddell, Robert Scott, "A Greek-English Lexicon", at Perseus

2. Genesis, Henry George Liddell, Robert Scott, "A Greek-English Lexicon", at Perseus

3. Online Etymology Dictionary

4. Griffiths, William M.; Miller, Jeffrey H.; Suzuki, David T. et al., eds (2000)."Genetics and the Organism: Introduction". An Introduction to Genetic Analysis (7th ed.). New York: W. H. Freeman. ISBN 0-7167-3520-2.

5. Hartl D, Jones E (2005)

6. Weiling, F (1991). "Historical study: Johann Gregor Mendel 1822–1884.".American journal of medical

genetics 40 (1): 1–25; discussion 26.doi:10.1002/ajmg.1320400103. PMID 1887835.

7. Lamarck, J-B (2008). In Encyclopædia Britannica. Retrieved fromEncyclopædia Britannica Online on 16 March 2008.

8. Peter J. Bowler, The Mendelian Revolution: The Emergency of Hereditarian Concepts in Modern Science and Society (Baltimore: Johns Hopkins University Press, 1989): chapters 2 & 3.

9. a b Blumberg, Roger B.. "Mendel's Paper in English".

10. genetics, n., Oxford English Dictionary, 3rd ed.

11. Bateson W. "Letter from William Bateson to Alan Sedgwick in 1905". The John Innes Centre. Retrieved 15 March 2008.. Note that the letter was to an Adam Sedgwick, a zoologist at Trinity College, Cambridge, not "Alan", and not to be confused with the renowned British geologist, Adam Sedgwick, who lived some time earlier.

12. genetic, adj., Oxford English Dictionary, 3rd ed.

13. Bateson, W (1907). "The Progress of Genetic Research". In Wilks, W.Report of the Third 1906 International Conference on Genetics: Hybridization (the cross-breeding of genera or species), the cross-breeding of varieties, and general plant breeding. London: Royal Horticultural Society.

Initially titled the "International Conference on Hybridisation and Plant Breeding", Wilks changed the title for publication as a result of Bateson's speech.[citation needed]

14. Moore, John A. (1983). "Thomas Hunt Morgan—The Geneticist". Integrative and Comparative Biology 23: 855. doi:10.1093/icb/23.4.855.

15. Sturtevant AH (1913). "The linear arrangement of six sex-linked factors in Drosophila, as shown by their mode of association". Journal of Experimental Biology 14: 43–59.

16. Avery, OT; MacLeod, CM; McCarty, M (1944). "STUDIES ON THE CHEMICAL NATURE OF THE SUBSTANCE INDUCING TRANSFORMATION OF PNEUMOCOCCAL TYPES : INDUCTION OF TRANSFORMATION BY A DESOXYRIBONUCLEIC

ACID FRACTION ISOLATED FROM PNEUMOCOCCUS TYPE III.". The Journal of experimental medicine 79 (2): 137–58. doi:10.1084/jem.79.2.137. PMID 19871359. Reprint: Avery, OT; Macleod, CM; Mccarty, M (1979). "Studies on the chemical nature of the substance inducing transformation of pneumococcal types. Inductions of transformation by a desoxyribonucleic acid fraction isolated from pneumococcus type III.". The Journal of experimental medicine 149 (2): 297–326. doi:10.1084/jem.149.2.297. PMID 33226.

17. Hershey, AD; Chase, M (1952). "Independent functions of viral protein and nucleic acid in growth of bacteriophage". The Journal of general physiology 36 (1): 39–56. doi:10.1085/jgp.36.1.39. PMID 12981234.

18. Judson, Horace (1979). The Eighth Day of Creation: Makers of the Revolution in Biology. Cold Spring Harbor Laboratory Press. pp. 51–169. ISBN 0-87969-477-7.

19. Watson, J. D.; Crick, FH (1953). "Molecular Structure of Nucleic Acids: A Structure for Deoxyribose Nucleic Acid". Nature 171 (4356): 737. doi:10.1038/171737a0. PMID 13054692.

20. Watson, J. D.; Crick, FH (1953). "Genetical Implications of the Structure of Deoxyribonucleic Acid". Nature 171 (4361): 964. doi:10.1038/171964b0.PMID 13063483.

21. Sanger, F; Nicklen, S; Coulson, AR (1977). "DNA sequencing with chain-terminating inhibitors". Proceedings of the National Academy of Sciences of the United States of America 74 (12): 5463–7.doi:10.1073/pnas.74.12.5463. PMID 271968.

22. Saiki, RK; Scharf, S; Faloona, F; Mullis, KB; Horn, GT; Erlich, HA; Arnheim, N (1985). "Enzymatic amplification of beta-globin genomic sequences and restriction site analysis for diagnosis of sickle cell anemia.". Science 230(4732): 1350–4. doi:10.1126/science.2999980. PMID 2999980.

23. a b "Human Genome Project Information". Human Genome Project. Retrieved 15 March 2008.

24. Griffiths, William M.; Miller, Jeffrey H.; Suzuki, David T. et al., eds (2000)."Patterns of Inheritance: Introduction". An Introduction to Genetic Analysis(7th ed.). New York: W. H. Freeman. ISBN 0-7167-3520-2.

25. Griffiths, William M.; Miller, Jeffrey H.; Suzuki, David T. et al., eds (2000)."Mendel's experiments". An Introduction to Genetic Analysis (7th ed.). New York: W. H. Freeman. ISBN 0-7167-3520-2.

26. a b c Griffiths, William M.; Miller, Jeffrey H.; Suzuki, David T. et al., eds (2000)."Mendelian genetics in eukaryotic life cycles". An Introduction to Genetic Analysis (7th ed.). New York: W. H. Freeman. ISBN 0-7167-3520-2.

27. Griffiths, William M.; Miller, Jeffrey H.; Suzuki, David T. et al., eds (2000)."Interactions between the alleles of one gene". An Introduction to Genetic Analysis (7th ed.). New York: W. H. Freeman. ISBN 0-7167-3520-2.

28. Cheney, Richard W.. "Genetic Notation". Retrieved 18 March 2008.

29. Griffiths, William M.; Miller, Jeffrey H.; Suzuki, David T. et al., eds (2000)."Human Genetics". An Introduction to Genetic Analysis (7th ed.). New York: W. H. Freeman. ISBN 0-7167-3520-2.

30. Griffiths, William M.; Miller, Jeffrey H.; Suzuki, David T. et al., eds (2000)."Gene interaction and modified dihybrid ratios". An Introduction to Genetic

Analysis (7th ed.). New York: W. H. Freeman. ISBN 0-7167-3520-2.

31. Mayeux, R (2005). "Mapping the new frontier: complex genetic disorders.".The Journal of clinical investigation 115 (6): 1404–7.doi:10.1172/JCI25421. PMID 15931374.

32. Griffiths, William M.; Miller, Jeffrey H.; Suzuki, David T. et al., eds (2000)."Quantifying heritability". An Introduction to Genetic Analysis (7th ed.). New York: W. H. Freeman. ISBN 0-7167-3520-2.

33. Luke, A; Guo, X; Adeyemo, AA; Wilks, R; Forrester, T; Lowe W, W; Comuzzie, AG; Martin, LJ et al. (2001). "Heritability of obesity-related traits among Nigerians, Jamaicans and US black people.". International journal of obesity and related metabolic disorders 25 (7): 1034–41.doi:10.1038/sj.ijo.0801650. PMID 11443503.

34. Pearson, H (2006). "Genetics: what is a gene?". Nature 441 (7092): 398–401. doi:10.1038/441398a. PMID 16724031.

35. Prescott, L (1993). Microbiology. Wm. C. Brown Publishers.ISBN 0697013723.

36. Griffiths, William M.; Miller, Jeffrey H.; Suzuki, David T. et al., eds (2000)."Mechanism of DNA Replication". An Introduction to Genetic Analysis (7th ed.). New York: W. H. Freeman. ISBN 0-7167-3520-2.

37. Gregory, SG; Barlow, KF; Mclay, KE; Kaul, R; Swarbreck, D; Dunham, A; Scott, CE; Howe, KL et al. (2006). "The DNA sequence and biological annotation of human chromosome 1.". Nature 441 (7091): 315–21.doi:10.1038/nature04727. PMID 16710414.

38. Alberts et al. (2002), II.4. DNA and chromosomes: Chromosomal DNA and Its Packaging in the Chromatin Fiber

39. Griffiths, William M.; Miller, Jeffrey H.; Suzuki, David T. et al., eds (2000). "Sex chromosomes and sex-linked inheritance". An Introduction to Genetic Analysis (7th ed.). New York: W. H. Freeman. ISBN 0-7167-3520-2.

40. Griffiths, William M.; Miller, Jeffrey H.; Suzuki, David T. et al., eds (2000)."Bacterial conjugation". An Introduction to Genetic Analysis (7th ed.). New York: W. H. Freeman. ISBN 0-7167-3520-2.

41. Griffiths, William M.; Miller, Jeffrey H.; Suzuki, David T. et al., eds (2000)."Bacterial transformation". An Introduction to Genetic Analysis (7th ed.). New York: W. H. Freeman. ISBN 0-7167-3520-2.

42. Griffiths, William M.; Miller, Jeffrey H.; Suzuki, David T. et al., eds (2000)."Nature of crossing-over". An Introduction to Genetic Analysis (7th ed.). New York: W. H. Freeman. ISBN 0-7167-3520-2.

43. Griffiths, William M.; Miller, Jeffrey H.; Suzuki, David T. et al., eds (2000)."Linkage maps". An Introduction to Genetic Analysis (7th ed.). New York: W. H. Freeman. ISBN 0-7167-3520-2.

44. Berg JM, Tymoczko JL, Stryer L, Clarke ND (2002). "I. 5. DNA, RNA, and the Flow of Genetic Information: Amino Acids Are Encoded by Groups of Three Bases Starting from a Fixed Point". Biochemistry (5th ed.). New York: W. H. Freeman and Company.

45. Crick, F (1970). "Central dogma of molecular biology.". Nature 227(5258): 561–3. doi:10.1038/227561a0. PMID 4913914.

46. Alberts et al. (2002), I.3. Proteins: The Shape and Structure of Proteins

47. Alberts et al. (2002), I.3. Proteins: Protein Function

48. "How Does Sickle Cell Cause Disease?". Brigham and Women's Hospital: Information Center for Sickle Cell and Thalassemic Disorders. 11 April 2002. Retrieved 23 July 2007.

49. Imes, DL; Geary, LA; Grahn, RA; Lyons, LA (2006). "Albinism in the domestic cat (Felis catus) is associated with a tyrosinase (TYR) mutation.".Animal genetics 37 (2): 175–8. doi:10.1111/j.1365-2052.2005.01409.x.PMID 16573534.

50. "MedlinePlus: Phenylketonuria". NIH: National Library of Medicine. Retrieved 15 March 2008.

51. Rosenthal, David (1964). The Genain quadruplets; a case study and theoretical analysis of heredity and environment in schizophrenia.. New York: Basic Books. ISBN B0000CM68F.

52. Brivanlou, AH; Darnell Je, JE (2002). "Signal transduction and the control of gene expression.". Science

295 (5556): 813–8.doi:10.1126/science.1066355. PMID 11823631.

53. Alberts et al. (2002), II.3. Control of Gene Expression – The Tryptophan Repressor Is a Simple Switch That Turns Genes On and Off in Bacteria

54. Jaenisch, R; Bird, A (2003). "Epigenetic regulation of gene expression: how the genome integrates intrinsic and environmental signals.". Nature genetics 33 Suppl: 245–54. doi:10.1038/ng1089. PMID 12610534.

55. Chandler, VL (2007). "Paramutation: from maize to mice.". Cell 128 (4): 641–5. doi:10.1016/j.cell.2007.02.007. PMID 17320501.

56. Griffiths, William M.; Miller, Jeffrey H.; Suzuki, David T. et al., eds (2000)."Spontaneous mutations". An Introduction to Genetic Analysis (7th ed.). New York: W. H. Freeman. ISBN 0-7167-3520-2.

57. Freisinger, E; Grollman, AP; Miller, H; Kisker, C (2004). "Lesion (in)tolerance reveals insights into DNA replication fidelity.". The EMBO journal 23 (7): 1494–505. doi:10.1038/sj.emboj.7600158.PMID 15057282.

58. Griffiths, William M.; Miller, Jeffrey H.; Suzuki, David T. et al., eds (2000)."Induced mutations". An Introduction to Genetic Analysis (7th ed.). New York: W. H. Freeman. ISBN 0-7167-3520-2.

59. Griffiths, William M.; Miller, Jeffrey H.; Suzuki, David T. et al., eds (2000)."Chromosome Mutation I: Changes in Chromosome Structure: Introduction". An Introduction to Genetic Analysis (7th ed.). New York: W. H. Freeman. ISBN 0-7167-3520-2.

60. Sawyer, SA; Parsch, J; Zhang, Z; Hartl, DL (2007). "Prevalence of positive selection among nearly neutral amino acid replacements in Drosophila.".Proceedings of the National Academy of Sciences of the United States of America 104 (16): 6504–10. doi:10.1073/pnas.0701572104.PMID 17409186.

61. Griffiths, William M.; Miller, Jeffrey H.; Suzuki, David T. et al., eds (2000)."Variation and its modulation". An Introduction to Genetic Analysis (7th ed.). New York: W. H. Freeman. ISBN 0-7167-3520-2.

62. Griffiths, William M.; Miller, Jeffrey H.; Suzuki, David T. et al., eds (2000)."Selection". An

Introduction to Genetic Analysis (7th ed.). New York: W. H. Freeman. ISBN 0-7167-3520-2.

63. Griffiths, William M.; Miller, Jeffrey H.; Suzuki, David T. et al., eds (2000)."Random events". An Introduction to Genetic Analysis (7th ed.). New York: W. H. Freeman. ISBN 0-7167-3520-2.

64. Darwin, Charles (1859). On the Origin of Species (1st ed.). London: John Murray. pp. 1. ISBN 0801413192.. Related earlier ideas were acknowledged in Darwin, Charles (1861). On the Origin of Species (3rd ed.). London: John Murray. xiii. ISBN 0801413192.

65. Gavrilets, S (2003). "Perspective: models of speciation: what have we learned in 40 years?". Evolution; international journal of organic evolution 57(10): 2197–215. doi:10.1554/02-727. PMID 14628909.

66. Wolf, YI; Rogozin, IB; Grishin, NV; Koonin, EV (2002). "Genome trees and the tree of life.". Trends in genetics 18 (9): 472–9. doi:10.1016/S0168-9525(02)02744-0. PMID 12175808.

67. "The Use of Model Organisms in Instruction". University of Wisconsin: Wisconsin Outreach Research Modules. Retrieved 15 March 2008.

68. "NCBI: Genes and Disease". NIH: National Center for Biotechnology Information. Retrieved 15 March 2008.

69. Davey Smith, G; Ebrahim, S (2003). "'Mendelian randomization': can genetic epidemiology contribute to understanding environmental determinants of disease?". International journal of epidemiology 32 (1): 1–22.doi:10.1093/ije/dyg070. PMID 12689998.

70. "Pharmacogenetics Fact Sheet". NIH: National Institute of General Medical Sciences. Retrieved 15 March 2008.

71. Frank, SA (2004). "Genetic predisposition to cancer - insights from population genetics". Nature reviews. Genetics 5 (10): 764–72.doi:10.1038/nrg1450. PMID 15510167.

72. Strachan T, Read AP (1999). Human Molecular Genetics 2 (second ed.). John Wiley & Sons Inc..Chapter 18: Cancer Genetics

73. Lodish et al. (2000), Chapter 7: 7.1. DNA Cloning with Plasmid Vectors

74. Lodish et al. (2000), Chapter 7: 7.7. Polymerase Chain Reaction: An Alternative to Cloning

75. Brown TA (2002). "Section 2, Chapter 6: 6.1. The Methodology for DNA Sequencing". Genomes 2 (2nd ed.). Oxford: Bios. ISBN 1 85996 228 9.

76. Brown (2002), Section 2, Chapter 6: 6.2. Assembly of a Contiguous DNA Sequence

77. Service, RF (2006). "Gene sequencing. The race for the $1000 genome.".Science 311 (5767): 1544–6. doi:10.1126/science.311.5767.1544.PMID 16543431.

References

Alberts B, Johnson A, Lewis J, Raff M, Roberts K, and Walter P (2002).Molecular Biology of the Cell (4th ed.). New York: Garland Science. ISBN 0-8153-3218-1.

Griffiths, William M.; Miller, Jeffrey H.; Suzuki, David T. et al., eds (2000).An Introduction to Genetic Analysis (7th ed.). New York: W. H. Freeman.ISBN 0-7167-3520-2.

Hartl D, Jones E (2005). Genetics: Analysis of Genes and Genomes (6th ed.). Jones & Bartlett. ISBN 0-7637-1511-5.

Lodish H, Berk A, Zipursky LS, Matsudaira P, Baltimore D, and Darnell J (2000). Molecular Cell Biology (4th ed.). New York: Scientific American Books. ISBN 0-7167-3136-3.

Wikipedia. Genetics. Article Retrieved October 10th, 2010 from: http://en.wikipedia.org/wiki/Genetics.

Glossary of Medical Terms

Abnormal: Not normal. Deviating from the usual position, condition, structure or behavior. An abnormal growth could indicate a premalignant or malignant condition. In other words, an abnormal growth could indicate cancer

Acquired: An acquired condition is one that isn't present at birth. In other words, it is a condition that is not inherited.

Acute: A condition with an abrupt onset. A brain aneurism is said to be acute if it comes on suddenly. An acute condition could also describe an illness of short duration that rapidly progresses and requires urgent care.

Airway: The trachea. A method of preventing sensation, used to eliminate pain. The loss or prevention of pain, as caused by anesthesia.

Aneurysm or Aneurism: An abnormal blood-filled swelling of an artery or vein, resulting from a localized weakness in the wall of the vessel.

Angiography: A medical imaging technique in which an X-ray image is taken to visualize the inside of blood vessels and organs of the body, with particular interest in the arteries, veins and the heart chambers.

Artery: An efferent blood vessel from the heart, conveying blood away from the heart regardless of oxygenation status.

Autopsy : A dissection performed on a cadaver to find possible cause(s) of death. An after-the-fact examination, especially of the causes of a failure.

Berry aneurysm: An aneurism that looks like a berry. It usually happens where a cerebral artery leaves the circular artery at the base of the brain.

Blood pressure: The pressure exerted by the blood against the walls of the arteries and veins; it varies during the heartbeat cycle, and according to a person'sage, health and physical condition. The great majority of people who have serious conditions from high blood pressure suffer debilitating illness.

Brain: The control center of thecentral nervous system of an animal located in the skull which is responsible for perception,cognition, attention, memory, emotion, and action.

Brain aneurysm: See berry aneurysm.

Brain swelling: See: Cerebral edema .

Breathing: The act of respiration; a single instance of this.

Calcium: A mineral stored in the bones. Calcium is added to bones by osteoblasts and is removed osteoclasts. This mineral s essential for healthy bones and regulates muscle contraction, heart action, nervous system maintenance, and normal blood clotting. Food sources of calcium include dairy foods, some leafy green vegetables such as broccoli and collards, canned salmon, clams, oysters, calcium-fortified foods, and tofu.

Calcium channel blocker: A drug that blocks calcium from entering the heart and artery muscle, preventing narrowing of the arteries.

Cardiovascular: Relating to the circulatory system, that is the heart and blood vessels.

Catheter: small tube inserted into a body cavity to remove fluid, create an opening, distend a passageway or administer a drug

Cell: The basic unit of a living organism, surrounded by a cell membrane.

Cerebral: Of, or relating to the brain or cerebral cortex of the brain.

Cerebral aneurysm: See: Berry aneurysm.

Cholesterol: A sterollipid synthesized by the liver and transported in the bloodstream to the membranes of all animal cells; it plays a central role in many biochemical processes and, as a lipoprotein that coats the walls of blood vessels, is associated with cardiovascular disease.

Circle of Willis: An arterial circle at the base of the brain.
Circulation: The movement of the blood in the blood-vascular system, by which it is brought into close relations with almost every living elementary constituent.

Cocaine: . A stimulant narcotic in the form of a white powder that users generally self-administer by insufflationthrough the nose. Any derivative of cocaine. Extracted from the leaves of the coca scrub (Erythroxylon coca) indigenous to the Andean highlands of South America.

Coma: A state of sleep from which one may not wake up, usually induced by some form of trauma.

Compression (medicine): Pressing together. As in a compression fracture , nerve compression , or spinal cord compression.

Compression(embryology): To shorten in time.

Connective tissue: type of tissue found in animals whose main function is binding other tissue systems (such as muscle to skin) or organs and consists of the following three elements: cells, fibers and a ground substance (or extracellular matrix).

Contrast: Any substance, such as barium sulfate, used in radiography to increase thevisibility of internal structures

CT scan: Computerized tomography scan. Pictures of the body created by a computer where multiple X-ray imagesare turned into pictures on a screen.

Cysts: A pouch or sac without opening, usually membranous and containing morbid matter, which develops in one of the natural cavities or in the substance of an organ.

Dizziness: he state of being dizzy; the sensation of instability.

Doppler ultrasound: A type of ultrasound that detects and measures blood flow.

Ehlers-Danlos syndrome : A heritable disorder of connective tissue with easy bruising, joint hypermobility (loose joints), skin laxity, and weakness of tissues.

Emergency department: The department of a hospital that treats emergencies.

Extended family: a family consisting of parents and children, along with either grandparents, grandchildren, aunts or uncles etc.

Extremity: the most extreme or furthest point of something.

1. An extreme measure.

2. A hand or foot.

Genetic: (genetics) relating to genetics or genes. Caused by genes.

Groin: The long narrow depression of the human body that separates the trunk from the legs.

Headache : A pain or ache in the head.

Hemorrhage: A heavy release of blood within or from the body.

High blood pressure : Hypertension: a repeatedly elevated blood pressure exceeding 140 over 90 mmHg -- a systolic pressure above 140 with a diastolic pressure above 90.

Inheritance: The hereditary passing of biological attributes from ancestors to their offspring.

Interventional: Intervening, interfering or interceding with the intent of modifying the outcome. For example, an interventional radiologist .

Intracranial: f or pertaining to the brain or inside of the head. Within the cranium.

Kidney: an organ in the body that produces urine.

Lifetime risk: The risk of developing a particular disease or dying from that disease during your lifetime.

Long-term memory: Permanent storage, management, and retrieval of information for later use.

Lumbar: Related to the lower back or loin.

Lumbar puncture: A diagnostic and at times therapeutic procedure performed to collect a sample of cerebrospinal fluid for biochemical, microbiological, and cytological analysis, or rarely to relieve increased intracranialpressure.

Marfan syndrome: A genetic disorder of the connective tissue that causes defects in the heart valves and aorta. Characterized by abnormalities of the eyes, skeleton, and cardiovascular system.

Memory: 1. The ability to recover information about past events or knowledge. 2.The process of recovering information about past events or knowledge. 3. Cognitive reconstruction. The brain engages in a remarkable reshuffling process in an attempt to extract what is general and what is particular about each passing moment.

Migraine: Usually, periodic attacks of headaches on one or both sides of the head. These may be accompanied by nausea, vomiting, increased sensitivity of the eyes to light (photophobia), increased sensitivity to sound (phonophobia), dizziness , blurred vision, cognitive disturbances, and other symptoms. Some migraines do not include headache, and migraines may or may not be preceded by an aura.

MRI: Abbreviation and nickname for magnetic resonance imaging . For more information, see: Magnetic Resonance Imaging ; Paul C. Lauterbur ; Peter Mansfield .

Nausea: Nausea, is the urge to vomit. It can be brought by many causes including, systemic illnesses, such as influenza , medications, pain, and inner ear disease. When nausea and/or vomiting are persistent, or when they are accompanied by other severe symptoms such as abdominal pain , jaundice , fever, or bleeding, a physician should be consulted.

Neck: The part of the body joining the head to the shoulders. Also, any narrow or constricted part of a bone or organ that joins its parts as, for example, the neck of the femur bone.

Nerve: A bundle of fibers that uses chemical and electrical signals to transmit sensory and motor information from one body part to another. See: Nervous system .

Nerve cell: See: Neuron .

Neurofibromatosis: A genetic disorder of the nervous system that primarily affects the development and growth of neural (nerve) cell tissues, causes tumors to grow on nerves, and may produce other abnormalities.

Neurological: Having to do with the nerves or the nervous system.

Neurology: The medical specialty concerned with the diagnosis and treatment of disorders of the nervous system -- the brain, the spinal cord, and the nerves.

Neuroradiology: The field within radiology that specializes in the use of radioactive substances, x-rays and scanning devices for the diagnosis and treatment of diseases of the nervous system. Neuroradiology involves the clinical imaging, therapy, and basic science of the central and peripheral nervous system , including but not limited to the brain, spine , head and neck , interventional procedures, techniques in imaging and intervention , and related educational, socioeconomic, and medicolegal issues.

Neurosurgeon: A physician trained in surgery of the nervous system and who specializes in surgery on the brain and other parts of the nervous system. Sometimes called a "brain surgeon."

NIH: The National Institutes of Health. The NIH is an important U.S. health agency. It is devoted to medical research. Administratively under the Department of Health and Human Services (HHS), the NIH consists of 20-some separate Institutes and Centers. NIH's program activities are represented by these Institutes and Centers.

Onset: In medicine, the first appearance of the signs or symptoms of an illness as, for example, the onset of rheumatoid arthritis . There is always an onset to a disease but never to the return to good health. The default setting is good health.

Outpatient: A patient who is not an inpatient (not hospitalized) but instead is cared for elsewhere -- as in a doctor's office, clinic, or day surgery center. The term outpatient dates back at least to 1715. Outpatient care today is also called ambulatory care.

Pain: An unpleasant sensation that can range from mild, localized discomfort to agony. Pain has both physical and emotional components. The physical part of pain results from nerve stimulation. Pain may be contained to a discrete area, as in an injury, or it can be more diffuse, as in disorders like fibromyalgia . Pain is mediated by specific nerve fibers that carry the pain impulses to the brain where their conscious appreciation may be modified by many factors.

Pharmacy: A location where prescription drugs are sold. A pharmacy is, by law, constantly supervised by a licensed pharmacist.

Polycystic kidney disease: One of the genetic disorders characterized by the development of innumerable cysts in the kidneys. These cysts are filled with fluid, and replace much of the mass of the kidneys. This reduces kidney function, leading to kidney failure.

Pupil: The opening of the iris. The pupil may appear to open (dilate) and close (constrict) but it is really the iris that is the prime mover; the pupil is merely the absence of iris. The pupil determines how much light is let into the eye. Both pupils are usually of equal size. If they are not, that is termed anisocoria (from "a-", not + "iso", equal + "kore", pupil = not equal pupils).

Radiologic: Having to do with radiology.

Radiologist: A physician specialized in radiology, the branch of medicine that uses ionizing and nonionizing radiation for the diagnosis and treatment of disease.

Residual: Something left behind. With residual disease, the disease has not been eradicated.

Risk factor: Something that increases a person's chances of developing a disease.

Rupture: A break or tear in any organ (such as the spleen) or soft tissue (such as the achilles tendon). Rupture of the appendix is more likely among uninsured and minority children when they develop appendicitis.

Saccular: From the Latin "sacculus" meaning a small pouch. As for example the alveolar saccules (little air pouches) within the lungs.

Saccular aneurysm: An aneurysm that resembles a small sack. A berry aneurysm is typically saccular. An aneurysm is a localized widening (dilatation) of an artery, vein, or the heart. At the area of an aneurysm, there is typically a bulge and the wall is weakened and may rupture. The word "aneurysm" comes from the Greek "aneurysma" meaning "a widening."

Scan: As a noun, the data or image obtained from the examination of organs or regions of the body by gathering information with a sensing device.

Seizure: Uncontrolled electrical activity in the brain, which may produce a physical convulsion, minor physical signs, thought disturbances, or a combination of symptoms.

Sensitivity: 1. In psychology, the quality of being sensitive. As, for example, sensitivity training, training in small groups to develop a sensitive awareness and understanding of oneself and of ones relationships with others. 2. In disease epidemiology, the ability of a system to detect epidemics and other changes in disease occurrence. 3. In screening for a disease, the proportion of persons with the disease who are correctly identified by a screening test. 4. In the definition of a disease, the proportion of persons with the disease who are correctly identified by defined criteria.

Skull: The skull is a collection of bones which encase the brain and give form to the head and face. The bones of the skull include the following: the frontal, parietal, occipital, temporal, sphenoid, ethmoid, zygomatic, maxilla, nasal, vomer, palatine, inferior concha, and mandible.

Spasm: A brief, automatic jerking movement. A muscle spasm can be quite painful, with the muscle clenching tightly. A spasm of the coronary artery can cause angina . Spasms in various types of tissue may be caused by stress, medication, over-exercise, or other factors.

Spinal cord: The major column of nerve tissue that is connected to the brain and lies within the vertebral canal and from which the spinal nerves emerge. Thirty-one pairs of spinal nerves originate in the spinal cord: 8 cervical , 12 thoracic , 5 lumbar, 5 sacral, and 1 coccygeal. The spinal cord and the brain constitute the central nervous system (CNS). The spinal cord consists of nerve fibers that transmit impulses to and from the brain. Like the brain, the spinal cord is covered by three connective-tissue envelopes called the meninges . The space between the outer and middle envelopes is filled with cerebrospinal fluid (CSF), a clear colorless fluid that cushions the spinal cord against jarring shock. Also known simply as the cord.

Spinal tap: Also known as a lumbar puncture or "LP", a spinal tap is a procedure whereby spinal fluid is removed from the spinal canal for the purpose of diagnostic testing. It is particularly helpful in the diagnosis of inflammatory diseases of the central nervous system, especially infections, such as meningitis. It can also provide clues to the diagnosis of stroke, spinal cord tumor and cancer in the central nervous system.

Stress: Forces from the outside world impinging on the individual. Stress is a normal part of life that can help us learn and grow. Conversely, stress can cause us significant problems.

Stroke: The sudden death of some brain cells due to a lack of oxygen when the blood flow to the brain is impaired by blockage or rupture of an artery to the brain. A stroke is also called a cerebrovascular accident or, for short, a CVA.

Subarachnoid: Literally, beneath the arachnoid, the middle of three membranes that cover the central nervous system. In practice, subarachnoid usually refers to the space between the arachnoid and the pia mater, the innermost membrane surrounding the central nervous system.

Subarachnoid hemorrhage: Bleeding within the head into the space between two membranes that surround the brain. The bleeding is beneath the arachnoid membrane and just above the pia mater. (The arachnoid is the middle of three membranes around the brain while the pia mater is the innermost one.)

Surgery: The word "surgery" has multiple meanings. It is the branch of medicine concerned with diseases and conditions which require or are amenable to operative procedures. Surgery is the work done by a surgeon. By analogy, the work of an editor wielding his pen as a scalpel is s form of surgery. A surgery in England (and some other countries) is a physician's or dentist's office.

Swelling of the brain: See: Cerebral edema .

Symptom: Any subjective evidence of disease. Anxiety, lower back pain , and fatigue are all symptoms. They are sensations only the patient can perceive. In contrast, a sign is objective evidence of disease. A bloody nose is a sign. It is evident to the patient, doctor, nurse and other observers.

Syndrome: A set of signs and symptoms that tend to occur together and which reflect the presence of a particular disease or an increased chance of developing a particular disease.

Temple: An area just behind and to the side of the forehead and the eye, above the side of the check bone (the zygomatic arch) and in front of the ear.

Tension: 1) The pressure within a vessel , such as blood pressure : the pressure within the blood vessels. For example, elevated blood pressure is referred to as hypertension . 2) Stress, especially stress that is translated into clenched scalp muscles and bottled-up emotions or anxiety. This is the type of tension blamed for tension headaches.

Therapeutic: Relating to therapeutics , that part of medicine concerned specifically with the treatment of disease . The therapeutic dose of a drug is the amount needed to treat a disease.

Throat: The throat is the anterior (front) portion of the neck beginning at the back of the mouth , consisting anatomically of the pharynx and larynx . The throat contains the trachea and a portion of the esophagus .

Tobacco: A South American herb, formally known as Nicotiana tabacum , whose leaves contain 2-8% nicotine and serve as the source of smoking and smokeless tobacco .

Transcranial: Through the cranium . As, for example, in transcranial magnetic stimulation .

Ultrasound : High-frequency sound waves. Ultrasound waves can be bounced off of tissues using special devices. The echoes are then converted into a picture called a sonogram. Ultrasound imaging, referred to as ultrasonography, allows physicians and patients to get an inside view of soft tissues and body cavities, without using invasive techniques. Ultrasound is often used to examine a fetus during pregnancy There is no convincing evidence for any danger from ultrasound during pregnancy.

Vessel: A tube in the body that carries fluids: blood vessels or lymph vessels.

Visual field: The entire area that can be seen when the eye is directed forward, including that which is seen with peripheral vision.

X-ray: 1. High-energy radiation with waves shorter than those of visible light. X-rays possess the properties of penetrating most substances (to varying extents), of acting on a photographic film or plate (permitting radiography), and of causing a fluorescent screen to give off light (permitting fluoroscopy). In low doses X-rays are used for making images that help to diagnose disease, and in high doses to treat cancer . Formerly called a Roentgen ray. 2. An image obtained by means of X-rays.

Appendix A: Internet Resources / Further Reading

The following Internet resources may be helpful in answering any health or medical questions you may have. The sites were chose because of their superior content, accuracy, and authority.

Print Publications Online

American Family Physician

http://www.aafp.org/online/en/home/publications/journals/afp.html
A full-text, online version of the esteemed journal. Contains excellent review articles on clinical medicine. Many come with patient education information.

Merck Manual of Diagnosis and Therapy, 17th ed.

http://www.merck.com/mmpe/index.html

A medical guide for professionals, available online. Contains technical information for a host of diseases along with their corresponding diagnosis an treatment suggestions.

Merck Manual of Geriatrics

http://www.merck.com/mkgr/mmg/home.jsp

Similar in format to the Merck Manual of Diagnosis and Therapy, this guide focuses on disorders and diseases with a slant towards implications for the elderly.

Merck Manual of Medical Information - 2nd Home Edition

http://www.merck.com/mmhe/index.html

A consumers' guide to diseases and their treatments. This is a complete online version of the text edition, with videos and a pronunciation guide

Postgraduate Medicine

http://www.postgradmed.com/

Professional medical journal with review articles on diseases and treatments. Although this is directed to the professional, the journal includes patient notes which are directed toward the general consumer.

MEDLINE/MedlinePlus

MEDLINE Plus

http://www.nlm.nih.gov/medlineplus/

Anatomy videos aimed at the general consumer plus thousands of articles on a variety of health related topics.

PubMed

http://www.ncbi.nlm.nih.gov/sites/entrez

PubMed comprises more than 20 million citations for biomedical literature from MEDLINE, life science journals, and online books. Citations may include links to full-text content from PubMed Central and publisher web sites.

NEWS SERVICES

These sources offer reliable information and up to date news stories about medical research.

Understanding Medical News

Consumer's Guide to Taking Charge of Medical Information

http://www.health-insight-harvard.org/

This guide, developed by the Harvard School of Public Health, helps you to decipher "scary" headlines.

Deciphering Medspeak

http://mlanet.org/resources/medspeak/index.html

To make informed health decisions, you have probably read a newspaper or magazine article, tuned into a radio or television program, or searched the Internet to find answers to health questions. If so, you have probably encountered "medspeak," the specialized language of health professionals. The Medical Library Association developed "Deciphering Medspeak" to help translate common "medspeak" terms.

HealthNewsReviews

http://www.healthnewsreview.org/

HealthNewsReview.org is a website dedicated to:
- Improving the accuracy of news stories about medical treatments, tests, products and procedures.
- Helping consumers evaluate the evidence for and against new ideas in health care.

Interpreting News on Diet and Nutrition

http://www.hsph.harvard.edu/nutritionsource/nutrition-news/media/

Confused by all the conflicting stories about what's good to eat and what's not? Sensational headlines don't always tell the whole story. Look at how nutrition news fits into the bigger scientific picture.

.

Understanding Risk. What Do Those Headlines Really Mean?

http://www.niapublications.org/tipsheets/pdf/Understanding_Risk-What_Do_Those_Headlines_Really_Mean.pdf

Tipsheet that discusses the differences among types of clinical research and explains the significance of types of risk in research results. Excellent easy to understand information about risk.

Beyond the Headlines: What Consumers Need To Know About Nutrition News

http://www.foodinsight.org/

The International Food Information Council Foundation is dedicated to the mission of effectively communicating science-based information on health, food safety and nutrition for the public good.

Recommended Online News Sources

Aetna InteliHealth Health News

http://www.intelihealth.com/IH/ihtIH/WSIHW000/333/333.html?k=menux408x333

Top news headlines for the day. T there is a section with commentaries written by Harvard Medical School physicians of several of the day's top news stories.

CNN Health

http://www.cnn.com/HEALTH/

Daily updated articles from a variety of news sources with links to related CNN stories and websites.

1st Headlines - Top Health Headlines

http://www.1stheadlines.com/health.htm

Top news stories from a variety of sources. Story may be covered by more than one news sources, allowing you to compare stories and fill in information gaps.

Reuters Health eLine

http://www.reutershealth.com/en/index.html

Daily medical news for the consumer (free) and for the professional (requires a subscription fee).

News Sources With Daily/Weekly Email Delivery

MedlinePlus Health News

http://www.nlm.nih.gov/medlineplus/

Produced by the National Library of Medicine, this site has daily news releases from sources such as United Press International, New York Times Syndicate, and Reuters. Stories can be retrieved for thirty days from publication. Users may sign up for daily email of "Health Headlines" in several different categories.

Medscape

http://www.medscape.com/

From WebMD, a website for doctors with a comprehensive news feature. Go to the website to read the daily news or sign
up for any of the forty free newsletters for delivery to your email address. There are newsletters in twenty-five specialties,
a weekly multi-specialty edition, health business news, and much more.

NewsWise

http://feeds.feedburner.com/NewswiseMednews

Medical news stories. Information from news releases of more than four hundred universities, professional associations, and research institutions. Register and sign up to receive weekly medical news digests via email.

Alternative Medicine**Ask Dr. Weil**

http://www.drweil.com/

The popular doctor discusses alternative healing remedies for many common ailments.

Alternative Medicine Homepage

http://www.pitt.edu/~cbw/altm.html
From the Falk Library of the Health Sciences, University of Pittsburgh - a jumpstation for sources of information on unconventional, alternative, complementary, innovative, and integrative therapies.

HerbMed

http://www.herbmed.org/

HerbMed is an interactive, electronic herbal database. It provides hyperlinked access to the scientific & medical research articles on the use of herbs for treating medical conditions. This evidence-based information resource is for professionals, researchers, and the general public.

National Center for Complementary and Alternative Medicine

http://nccam.nih.gov/

General information about alternative and complementary therapies with links to research studies currently being conducted on alternative therapies for a variety of conditions.

Rosenthal Center for Complementary and Alternative Medicine

http://www.rosenthal.hs.columbia.edu//

Links to resources on acupuncture, homeopathy, chiropractic, and herbal medicine and alternative therapies for cancer and women's health. The Center sponsors research on alternative and complementary medical practices.

CLINICAL RESEARCH TRIALS

Center Watch

http://www.centerwatch.com/

Information on over 41,000 clinical trials for twenty disease categories. Profiles of 150 research centers conducting clinical trials and profiles of companies that provide a variety of contract services to the clinical trials industry. Includes industry and government sponsored clinical trials and information on new drug treatments approved by the Food and Drug Administration.

Clinical Trials

http://www.clinicaltrials.gov/

Information on current research being conducted on treatments for different diseases. Browse by disease category and sponsor or search the entire site. Learn what clinical trials are all about and how to decide to participate in a trial.

DISEASES, MEDICAL CONDITIONS, GENERAL HEALTH

Aetna Intelihealth

http://www.intellihealth.com/IH/ihtIH?t=408

From the Harvard Medical School, information on diseases and medical conditions, health and fitness, medications, nutrition,
childbirth, and other topics.

Healthfinder

http://www.healthfinder.gov/

From the U.S. Department of Health and Human Services, a gateway to consumer information on diseases, medical conditions,
health promotion, and many other topics.

Mayo Clinic
http://www.mayoclinic.com/

From the famed Mayo Clinic, information on diseases and conditions, treatment decisions, drugs and supplements, healthy living,
and health assessment tools. Special features include online videos of exercises, diagnostic tests, surgical procedures, and medical conditions, healthy recipes, and self-care information.

National Organization for Rare Diseases

http://www.rarediseases.org/

Basic information on rare diseases and disorders. Full-reports are available for a fee.

NOAH (New York Online Access to Health)

http://www.noah-health.org/
English and Spanish language information and resources from organizations and governmental agencies. Aging, cancer, asthma, eye diseases, foot and ankle disorders, and pain are just a few of the topics covered.

HEALTH CARE PROVIDERS

American Board of Medical Specialties (ABMS)

http://www.abms.org/

Verify the certification status of any physician in the 24 specialities of the ABMS. Registration is required (free) and user is limited to five searches in a 24 hour period.

AMA Physician Select

https://extapps.ama-assn.org/doctorfinder/recaptcha.jsp

Gives credentials of MD's and DO's including medical school, year of graduation, and specialties.

American Hospital Directory

http://www.ahd.com/
Profiles of U.S. hospitals. Basic service is free; more detailed information by paid subscription only.

Federation of State Medical Boards

http://www.fsmb.org/

Select "Public Services" from the left-hand index, then select "Directory of State Medical Boards" to find links to web sites for the 50 U.S. States, plus the District of Columbia, Guam, and the Northern Mariana Islands. Not all of the states have physician profile or disciplinary action information. There are also links to osteopathic physician sites when available.

Health Pages

http://www.healthpages.com/

Information about physicians, dentists, hospitals and clinics, elder care facilities, dietitians and nutritionists.

Joint Commission on the Accreditation of Healthcare Organizations

http://www.jointcommission.org/

The Quality Check feature on this site supplies details on individual hospital performance ratings from JCAHO's accreditation reports. View Performance Reports and compare institutions' ratings. Reports cover hospitals, nursing homes, ambulatory care facilities, home care, laboratory services, and long term care facilities.

Nursing Home Compare

http://www.medicare.gov/NHCompare/Include/DataSection/Questions/SearchCriteriaNEW.asp?version=default&browser=Chrome|6|WinNT&language=English&defaultstatus=0&pagelist=Home&CookiesEnabledStatus=True

Provides detailed information about the performance of every Medicare and Medicaid certified nursing home in the country. Searchable by state. Includes a guide to choosing a nursing home and a nursing home checklist to help in making informed choices.

Questions and Answers About Health Insurance: A Consumer Guide

http://www.ahrq.gov/consumer/insuranceqa/

Questions and answers on choosing and using a health plan.

Quackery and Health Fraud**Quackwatch**

http://www.quackwatch.com/

Want information about whether those alternative therapies work? This site has information on health fraud, medical quackery, "new age" medicine and "alternative" and "complementary" medicine.

National Council Against Health Fraud

http://www.ncahf.org/
Non-profit voluntary health agency focusing on health fraud, misinformation, and quackery as public health concerns. Read their position papers on acupuncture, homepathy, chiropractic, and other health issues.

SURGERY

American College of Surgeons

http://www.facs.org/
   Public information section offers guidelines on choosing a qualified surgeon.

Tests and Procedures - MedlinePlus

http://www.nlm.nih.gov/medlineplus/tutorial.html
Interactive tutorials on 24 common tests and diagnostic procedures and more than 30 surgeries and treatment procedures.

Back to Contents

REFERENCES

Albert, G, Menezes, A. et al. (2010). Chiari Malformation Type I in Chidren Younger Than Age 6 Years. Journal of Neurosurgery. vol.5. number 6.

Columbia University Medical Center (2010). Medical First: Boy's Brainstem Saved by a Nose, Retrieved October 1st from http://www.columbianeurosurgery.org/2010/01/medical-first-boys-brainstem-saved-by-a-nose.

Columbia University Medical Center (2010). Chiari Malformation, Retrieved October 1st from http://www.columbianeurosurgery.org/conditions/chiari-malformation

Eule, J, Erickson, M. et al. (2002). Chiari I Malformation Associated with Syringomyelia and Scoliosis. SPINE. vol.27. number.13. pp. 1451:1455.

National Institute of Neurological Disorders and Stroke (2010). Chiari Malformation, Retrieved October 1st from http://www.ninds.nih.gov/disorders/chiari/detail_chiari.htm.

Piatt, J. (2004). The Chiari Malformation: What Does It Mean? Drexel University College of Medicine Pediatric Neurosurgery.

UCLA (2010). Chiari Malformatin, Retrieved October 1st from http://neurosurgery.ucla.edu/body.cfm?id=126.

Rueffner, K, RN (2010) Planning Brain Surgery. University of West Georgia. Article Retrieved October 4th, 2010 from http://stu.westga.edu/~wmaples/planning.html

Photographs

MRI Machine: Photographed by Wikimedia User:KasugaHuang on Mar 27, 2006 at Tri-Service General Hospital, Taiwan.

MRI of the brain: image courtesy of TheBrain|Wikimedia.org.

Head X-Ray by Mnolf|Wikimedia.org

Two hemisphere of the brain by Octavio L|Wikimedia.org

Amygdala by Washington Irving | Wikimedia.org

Midbrain by Hk kng|Wikimedia.org

Made in the USA
Lexington, KY
06 December 2012